ABOUT THE AUTHORS

YALE SOLOMON, M.D., began practicing ophthalmology in Bay Shore, New York, in 1956. Now retired from general ophthalmology, Dr. Solomon currently maintains a practice specializing in treating patients with macular degeneration and low vision. Earlier in his career, he was an associate clinical professor of ophthalmology at SUNY Stony Brook School of Medicine on Long Island, and he held senior positions in the ophthalmology departments at Southside Hospital in Bay Shore and Good Samaritan Hospital in West Islip, New York. He is also the founder and chairman of Volunteer Eye Surgeons International, a philanthropic organization that since 1986 has sent U.S. ophthalmologists to Third World countries on medical mercy missions. In 1990, at age 64, Dr. Solomon was diagnosed with macular degeneration in his left eye, and in the summer of 1997 macular degeneration began affecting vision in his right eye. Dr. Solomon lives in Huntington, New York, with his wife, Isobel. They have four grown sons and ten grandchildren.

JONATHAN D. SOLOMON is an independent marketing consultant and business writer. A graduate of Wesleyan University, Mr. Solomon also earned a Master of Science degree in journalism from Boston University and an MBA in marketing from Fordham University. He is the author of *The Tinen Killings* (BookSurge 2008), a novel of Civil War veterans. Mr. Solomon, who is Yale Solomon's oldest son, lives in Westfield, New Jersey, with his wife, Maureen, and their two children.

OVERCOMING MACULAR DEGENERATION

A GUIDE TO SEEING BEYOND THE CLOUDS

YALE SOLOMON, M.D.
With Jonathan D. Solomon

The information contained in Overcoming Macular Degeneration is not intended to replace the care prescribed by your physician. Always consult your physician before beginning a new health regimen or altering any course of treatment set up by your doctor.

Excerpt from "Monet Refuses the Operation" reprinted by permission of Louisiana State University Press from *Alive Together: New and Selected Poems* by Lisel Mueller. Copyright © 1996 by Lisel Mueller.

Cover design by Nadeem Zaidi, Mecca New York.
www.meccanewyork.com

BookSurge Publishing.

Visit www.amazon.com to order additional copies.

To Isobel
For boundless inspiration, exhortation,
and toleration, combined with even greater
assistance and—supreme value—infinite love.

—Y.S.

Doctor, you say there are no halos
around the streetlights in Paris
and what I see is an aberration
caused by old age, an affliction.
I tell you it has taken me all my life
to arrive at the vision of gas lamps as angels,
to soften and blur and finally banish
the edges you regret I don't see,
to learn that the line I called the horizon
does not exist and the sky and water,
so long apart, are the same state of being…

—Lisel Mueller, "Monet Refuses the Operation"

Contents

Contents

INTRODUCTION

You Are Not Alone

Like you, I am one of some ten to twenty million Americans with age-related macular degeneration. This disease, for which there is no cure, is the leading cause of severe visual impairment in this country, as it is in most other developed nations.

Each year, as many as 400,000 Americans are diagnosed with age-related macular degeneration, or AMD. The disease affects approximately one out of four people aged sixty-five or older. The surge in AMD cases over recent decades is an ironic side effect of medical progress and the longer life spans it has given us.

There are two types of age-related macular degeneration. Most AMD patients—about 90 percent—have the dry type, which takes years to progress and may never rob the patient of all central vision, although it certainly robs people of the retirement lifestyle they expected. The remaining 10 percent have the wet type, which leads to sudden and a much more severe loss of functional vision.

An AMD Patient and Physician

My own perspective on macular degeneration is somewhat special, for in addition to being an AMD patient, I am also an ophthalmologist. Over the years, I diagnosed hundreds of people with age-related macular degeneration. Now that my condition has stopped me from practicing general and surgical ophthalmology, I have devoted my practice exclusively to working with AMD patients. Here is my story.

I have always had a restless spirit. One thing that never varied, however, was the sense that I would be a physician. Two months after I was handed my U.S Army discharge papers after World War II, I was admitted into medical school as the youngest member of the class of 1950. My graduation was marked with some honor, including the award for psychiatry—a testament, I believe, to a capacity for empathy. My sense of adventure led me to become a ship's surgeon on the Grace Lines, and then into a general practice in a rural community.

My career in ophthalmology began when I joined an expatriate Texan who had started a practice on the then-rural eastern end of Long Island. Together we developed the largest private group of ophthalmologists in New York at the time.

When the medical school at the New York State University at Stony Brook was formed, I was asked to join as an associate clinical professor of ophthalmology. My ability to translate highly technical oph-thalmology concepts into language the students could understand led to several invitations, including one to write the chapters on ophthalmology in definitive medical textbooks in family practice and general medicine.

Some years later, when I learned through a medical mission group that the small island country of Saint Lucia in the Windward Islands of the Caribbean had no eye surgery available at its remote hospital, my curiosity spurred me to volunteer for a month as a visiting ophthalmologist. I found myself with the skills and expertise to effect the most magical change in individual lives. Straightening out a child's terribly crossed eyes, restoring vision to frail and elderly women and men blinded by neglected cataracts, and preventing glaucoma from progressing into blindness were wonderful accomplishments. That month left me profoundly changed, and I pursued other medical mercy assignments in the years that followed.

During one such mission to India in 1986 I realized the potential benefit of recruiting other like-minded eye surgeons for service in desperately needy areas. That concept became reality when I was able to raise sufficient funds from public and private sources to found an organization called Volunteer Eye Surgeons International. The purpose was to recruit ophthalmologists to teach and operate for a month in underdeveloped countries. Over the years we have sent eye surgeons to help in Vietnam, Thailand, India, Bangladesh, Java, New Guinea, Liberia, and Djibouti, among many other countries.

A Missing Fan Blade

My rather hectic pace involving international eye care and other interests was abruptly interrupted one morning when I observed something with my own eyes, in my own bedroom. The ceiling of my bedroom is painted a stark white. Hanging in the center is a fan, which on a cool October morning was not rotating. As I opened my eyes to greet a beautiful Sunday dawn, I noticed that the end of one blade was missing! Realizing that my right arm was lying over my closed right eye, I quickly un-covered my eye and was relieved to find that the fan was indeed whole again, with no defective blade.

A few seconds later my ophthalmologist brain shouted at me: "There's something seriously wrong here, stupid!" I then began a systematic process of self-examination. I proceeded silently to avoid disturbing my soundly sleeping wife, but I became increasingly aware of the pounding of my heart. Lying quietly, my face only inches from my wife's, I was aware of being alone in a rising cloud of fear.

I moved quickly to establish my diagnosis. Cover

left eye: fan totally clear and intact; cover right eye, focus on center of fan: end of one blade missing. End of case. Something very amiss with the edge of my macula. The diagnosis of a form of macular degeneration was confirmed that morning by my friend and ophthalmology associate Dr. Charles Beyrer.

A Search for Answers

As much as I respected and believed in my friend, a retina specialist with years of experience, I reacted the same as any patient facing vision loss. I went to be examined by super-experts in Baltimore, New York and Philadelphia. I desperately wanted someone to tell me that he or she had the potion to cure me, or at least preserve my good eye.

My encounters with a number of internationally respected retinologists are what really convinced me to write this book. I decided to counter the cool, unsympathetic attitude of some of the experts and to augment and affirm the supportive, warm reassurance of others. My own experience with these super-experts varied from a brusque, three-minute confirmation of the diagnosis to a supportive technical prognosis with compassionate responses to all my questions.

The realization that I, an experienced and knowledgeable ophthalmologist, could feel as lost and abandoned as I did upon learning my diagnosis led me to investigate what was available to inform the average intelligent, nonmedical man or woman with the same condition. What I discovered at the time was that a small number of worthy organizations have informative pamphlets or fliers about age-related macular degeneration. But there were no definitive books from "the inside." Nothing covered everything from the emotional reaction of the patient and family to careful explanations of the condition, including possible treatment, likely outcomes and specifics about rehabilitating one's life.

In the time since my initial diagnosis, I have found a unique role as a one-man consumer's advocate on the subject of macular degeneration. I could carefully evaluate low vision aids and devices by closing my good eye and determining the level of difficulty imposed by my central blind spot. I could judge the degree of benefit to be derived from various techniques and devices. There actually are many options available. In fact, I established a practice devoted to macular degeneration and the rehabilitation of low vision and lives affected by it. What I have learned through thirteen years of this clinical experience I hope to convey to you in this book.

The force that drives me to compile this material for you was greatly increased in 2004. On a bright and happy Fourth of July, an instantaneous blur in my central vision blasted the fact into my consciousness that my fairly good right eye had suddenly deteriorated from the mild, dry form of macular degeneration into the more serious wet form, caused by a leak from a small blood vessel into my macula. My sudden descent into legal blindness has emphasized for me three basic realizations:

1. **The initial diagnosis of macular degeneration has devastating implications for the patient.**

2. **At present, very little can be done to cure or improve macular degeneration.**

3. **Most ophthalmologists do not have the time, nor sometimes the inclination or compassion, to help the patient after making the diagnostic pronouncement.**

This book also sets three rather general goals:

1. **To help patients and families understand the nature and the natural course of the disease.**

2. **To reassure you that while at times you may feel hopeless and fear loss of independence, science offers great hope for overcoming visual impairments.**

3. **To enable patients to increase their visual ability to the maximum degree possible and thus achieve a satisfying life. This life may**

well be more difficult, but it can nevertheless be a rewarding and enjoyable one.

Let us now start the journey to seeing beyond the clouds.

CHAPTER 1

Diagnosis

Ophthalmologists are not very comfortable dealing with macular degeneration. Like most specialists, we prefer cases that have definitive solutions. Faced with an eye problem, we look for medicines, surgical procedures, or new laser treatments that can solve it. We gain our emotional rewards from improving people's vision.

Consider cataract surgery. A patient's vision is severely clouded. We operate. The patient sees normally again. For an eye doctor, what could be more gratifying?

Unfortunately, with macular degeneration there is no definitive medical or surgical solution. There are no drugs to prescribe, nor is there any routine operation to perform. Ophthalmologists can't cure macular degeneration, so they don't particularly like dealing with it.

A Brief Discussion Followed by Confusion

One reason so many patients are confused and concerned after learning from their ophthalmologist that they have macular degeneration is that the entire discussion about their condition and the future of their vision is usually brief. Indeed, most patients leave their ophthalmologist without a real understanding of the disease. They are left with many unanswered questions about what will happen to them and how they are going to cope with a progressive loss of sight.

Those patients who really tune in to what their ophthalmologist is saying during these short conversations will likely hear little more than these three key messages:

- You have macular degeneration. It is an age-related defect of the retina.

- There is really nothing we can do about it.

- Your vision may continue to deteriorate, but you are really not going to be blind.

If you are like most macular degeneration patients, that may have been the essence of the conversation that ended a process started some weeks earlier, with a decision to visit your ophthalmologist.

At the Beginning

You probably first noticed that you were having difficulty reading, especially in low light. Night driving was becoming harder. Letters may have appeared slightly distorted; perhaps door frames and other straight objects looked bent. While rubbing one eye you may have noticed that vision in the other was particularly blurry. It had gotten to the point where your vision problems were an ongoing annoyance that were interfering with some of your daily activities, so you made an appointment to see an ophthalmologist.

Actually, the onset of your macular degeneration most likely occurred months or even years earlier, particularly if it is worse in one eye than the other. Your good eye simply compensated for the bad one. If you think about it, you can probably recall some earlier vision problems, but none serious enough to warrant a visit to the doctor.

Don't be hard on yourself for not addressing the problem, and don't blame your eye care professional for not uncovering it earlier. Macular degeneration cannot easily be diagnosed during brief, routine eye exams, and anyway it isn't like cancer; early diagnosis has no bearing on the course of the most prevalent form of the disease, the dry form, nor does it open up additional treatment options.

If you are like some patients, you may have gone first to your optometrist. Or if you belong to an HMO, you may have seen your primary care doctor first. However, neither optometrists nor primary care physicians can easily or definitively diagnose macular degeneration, so you ended up visiting an ophthalmologist, a medical doctor who specializes in eye care.

What were your thoughts when you made that appointment? You probably assumed you just needed new glasses. Perhaps you suspected a cataract, which is the clouding of the eye's lens. Either way, you expected a neat solution: a prescription for new glasses or an appointment for cataract surgery, in which the clouded lens is removed from the eye and an artificial lens is inserted. Frankly, those would have been perfectly reasonable expectations. In fact, refractive changes, which are solved with new glasses, and cataracts are both far more common age-related causes of vision loss than macular degeneration. Indeed, they are the first two things your ophthalmologist looked for during your exam.

About Your Exam

The doctor almost certainly began your exam with general questions about your sight, and particularly about your overall health. This is because diabetes, high blood pressure, and other diseases also contribute to age-related vision loss. He or she also would have measured your vision and looked inside your eye with special devices such as ophthalmoscopes, biomicroscopes, and digital cameras. You were probably asked to use an Amsler grid card, which looks like a piece of graph paper. (See page 215. Macular degeneration patients tend to see the straight lines on the card as bent or wavy.)

With many patients, the steps in this kind of eye examination can lead to a conclusive diagnosis of macular degeneration. Some patients require more advanced testing and are sent to an ophthalmologist who specializes in the retina.

Let's digress briefly to discuss the role of the retina. There will be more detail about how the eye works in the chapters ahead, but here are the essential facts: The retina is a delicate layer of cells that lines the rear of the eye, on the inside. The lens of the eye, near the front, focuses images from the world onto the retina. The retina, in turn, transmits those images to the optic nerve. The optic nerve sends the images to the brain's sight center, which interprets them. The retina is like the film of a camera, and the macula is the bull's-eye of the retina. It is only as big as the head of a large pin, but the macula is the portion of the retina that is responsible for clear, central vision.

If you saw a retinal specialist, you probably had special pictures, called angiograms, taken of your retina, and you may have undergone other tests also. These other tests might have included visual field studies (measuring your side vision), high-power magnification studies of the macula conducted with a special contact lens and biomicroscope, contrast sensitivity testing (measuring your ability to discern shades of gray and other colors), color vision testing, ultrasonography (getting soundwave imagery of the eye), and the use of a device called a scanning laser ophthalmoscope to localize early macular changes. You may also have been examined with Optical Coherence Tomography, or OCT, which produces cross-section images of any part of the macula or retina. The angiograms and other tests were done to confirm your ophthalmologist's suspicions that you have macular degeneration and to determine what type of macular degeneration you have.

The Doctor-Patient Relationship

At this point, the doctor-patient relationship often becomes strained. There is no easy way for us as ophthalmologists to deliver the news to a patient that he or she has macular degeneration. Deep in his or her heart, the ophthalmologist knows that nothing can be done to reverse the loss of vision, and that the vision loss will probably continue. Meanwhile, in the waiting room outside, there are people with more readily treatable eye problems. So the patient gets the diagnosis and the quick speech about how his or her vision may deteriorate further and nothing can be done about it. The doctor will almost certainly offer words of encouragement about "not going blind." The patient may receive a little brochure about macular degeneration, and be urged to schedule a follow-up visit in six months so the doctor can monitor the progress of the disease.

Here is what generally does not happen in these conversations. The doctor usually does not take the time to explain the mechanics of sight and how vision is affected by macular degeneration. There is usually no discussion with the patient and his or her spouse or other caregiver about what kinds of lifestyle changes will become necessary. Often, the doctor doesn't even provide a referral to people or agencies that specialize in working with low-vision patients.

A Case Study

Let me tell you what happened with me. When I learned that I was developing macular degeneration, I made an appointment with an ophthalmologist who is a nationally known macula specialist at a major teaching hospital. After confirming my diagnosis he spoke with me for less than three minutes. I know—I looked at my watch. Keep in mind that I was a fellow ophthalmologist, and that I had referred patients to him over the years. But never once during those three minutes did he utter so much as a word of compassion for a colleague who had this disease.

For me, the message was clear: I'm a lost cause; my case is hopeless. I left in a fog of pessimism. Even just a few words of reassurance and support from this doctor would have gone a long way toward helping me feel a lot better.

Why, then, are so many of these conversations so cursory, so short? Why are they so lacking in empathy or practical advice? Don't we as ophthalmologists care about people with macular degeneration?

Of course we do. But many issues are at work.

Some of the blame can fairly be placed on today's great medical bogeyman, managed care. As doctors are pressured by the economics of managed care to see more patients in less time, patient education and bedside manner are suffering in all specialties.

That is only part of the answer, though. Another consideration is that doctors, after all, are only human, and it is difficult for one person to tell another bad news. This is particularly true for doctors because patients expect us to be all-knowing. An ophthalmologist finds it hard to look patients in the eye and tell them that they will probably lose most of their functional sight and that nothing can be done about it.

A practical reason for not immediately giving newly diagnosed patients an extensive education about macular degeneration is that they are often in a state of near shock upon learning about their condition and its implications. They may be in no condition to understand a lesson about the anatomy of the eye or a discussion about the physics of sight. Furthermore, a practical suggestion that they seek out an organization that specializes in helping people with limited vision could counter the much more important psychological message that "you won't go blind." For instance, a referral to Lighthouse International, which runs excellent programs for people with macular degeneration but which is also known as an institution for the blind, could be devastating to a newly diagnosed patient.

The most important factor behind these all-too-brief conversations, though, is that the patient suddenly stops needing an ophthalmologist and begins needing a counselor. And that is a role that ophthalmologists, by their training and experience, are unprepared to fill. Ophthalmologists are just not properly prepared to deal with these patients and their needs.

In my case, that macula specialist probably did consider me a lost cause. Despite all of his advanced training and years of experience, there really was nothing he could do for me medically or surgically. I knew that too, but it would have been nice to hear him extend some cause for optimism.

A Wish List

In an ideal world, a patient newly diagnosed with macular degeneration would be invited to return for a consultative visit, and to bring close family members to the session. That visit should happen within a week or two of the diagnosis, and should last at least twenty minutes. It would be a chance for the ophthalmologist to speak calmly with the patient, to answer questions and address concerns, and to provide referrals to resources that can help. By conducting such a session soon after, but not during, the initial visit, the ophthalmologist would avoid the difficulties of communicating with someone who has just received distressing news.

When I was practicing ophthalmology full-time I was probably as guilty of this doctor-patient transgression as many of my colleagues. I do remember, though, pulling apart my trusty model of the eyeball and pointing out to my patients the retina and the macula. I would talk about how there was a defect in the "film" of their eye, and how it was a common age-related condition, like hardening of the arteries. So maybe my conversations would last five or six minutes. My patients were probably still going home in more than a little psychological trouble.

Now that I am a patient with this disorder myself, I see firsthand the huge gap between what the typical ophthalmologist tells someone with macular degeneration and what the patient really wants and needs to know about the disease and its implications. Filling that gap is the purpose of the rest of this book.

CHAPTER 2

You Won't Need a Guide Dog

There is no person afflicted with age-related macular degeneration who has not experienced the grip of despair, even panic, at the thought of impending blindness. Even those, like myself, who *know* that blindness is a rare outcome from macular degeneration are not free from this despair. Why? Because the fear of blindness—no, *terror* at the thought of it—is virtually hardwired into our genes.

But now the good news: This won't happen to you. That's worth repeating.

You are not going to be blind. You're not going to need a guide dog or a cane. In no way. Never.

When most people imagine blindness they think about what their world would be like if their eyes were closed forever. But that is not what happens with macular degeneration.

Yes, your vision will deteriorate. In most cases—but not all—the impairment worsens over time, sometimes slowly and sometimes not. If you want to move forward with your life, you must understand that your vision will probably become diminished or distorted—certainly altered in ways that you couldn't imagine when everything was normal. But you are not going to go blind.

A poem by Lisel Mueller, "Monet Refuses the Operation," gave me new perspective on viewing things differently. Claude Monet, the great impressionist artist, developed increasingly severe cataracts and probably a form of macular degeneration. He initially did refuse to have surgery for his cataracts, and Mueller beautifully speculates on Monet's innermost thoughts. Read the opening of her poem as the epigraph of this book; her perspective on Monet's condition can truly alter our view of the effect of eye disease on us.

What Is Blindness, Anyway?

For the present, let us talk further about what is really meant by the medical use of the terms blindness and legal blindness. To an ophthalmologist, blindness means a patient has absolutely no perception of light. The world is dark. Again, this is not what happens to macular degeneration patients.

Legal blindness is a term that has been established for the purposes of compensation or disability determination. The general requirement for legal blindness is less than 20/200 vision in the better eye, or a visual field (side vision) of less than 20 degrees. (The normal field is usually 150 degrees wide.) Age-related macular degeneration (AMD) is the leading cause of legal blindness in America.

Most age-related macular degeneration patients have a normally wide field of vision, yet some may not be able to see the large E or 3 on eye-test charts from twenty feet away, and may therefore be classified as legally blind. While this level of impairment would certainly affect your lifestyle quite significantly, you would still not be blind. (You would, however, reap some financial benefits, such as income tax credits and free or reduced transit fares.)

Regrettably, many eye doctors use the term legally blind without realizing the full impact that this has on people. Often, eye doctors do early AMD patients great psychic harm by prematurely talking about legal blindness as a possible outcome of their condition.

Those with age-related macular degeneration should avoid dwelling on whether they are blind, functionally blind, or legally blind. Instead, they should focus on ways to maintain their lifestyle by learning to compensate for the loss of visual acuity. In order to do this, they must understand the changes in vision that occur because of age-related macular degeneration.

Understanding Early Symptoms

In the early stages of macular degeneration, vision is only minimally affected. If the condition is confined to one eye, as is often the case, the impairment is usually ignored because the good eye takes over. Therefore, unless the slight decrease in vision is specifically looked for, the patient rarely notices it.

One early manifestation of AMD that is recognized by most patients, however, involves the visual function of contrast sensitivity. The normal eye can discern more than the difference between extremes of shading, such as dense black against stark white; it also can pick out very fine differences, such as darker gray against slightly lighter gray. Many people with early macular degeneration notice a decrease in their contrast sensitivity. As a result, it becomes somewhat more difficult to read in dim light and to drive at night.

Interestingly, the patient's spouse rather than the patient himself or herself will often be the first to notice these early signs of visual difficulty. A frequent request to increase the lighting, a reluctance to drive after dark, or a sudden need to use a magnifier to read fine print may be early indications of macular degeneration.

At this stage, the changes in the eye's anatomy and function may be minimal, perhaps even undetectable except by sophisticated testing. Even routine eye examinations (which everyone over age sixty should have each year) might not uncover early stages of macular degeneration.

As the condition progresses, though, people become more aware of visual problems. Straight lines, such as flagpoles or doorways, may appear bent or wavy. Printed text may be distorted, or portions of words may appear to be missing. This is the point when most people realize they have a problem and schedule an eye exam. Typically, they think they simply need new glasses or, at worst, a cataract operation.

Other Age-Related Vision Problems

As noted in the previous chapter, these assumptions are not unreasonable. Indeed, most people who pick up a magnifying glass to verify a telephone number or stock quote do not necessarily have macular degeneration; in fact, they probably do not. Visual changes with aging are extremely common. For instance, normal changes in the lens of the eye that occur to everyone in their forties or fifties, a condition called presbyopia, results in increasing difficulty with reading, sewing, and other close-up tasks. Also, the lens of the eye tends to become more dense with age, which limits vision. Another age-related vision problem occurs when the size of the pupil, the round hole in the center of the iris through which light enters, decreases. These normal changes occur in a varying degree to all of us, and they are quite different from the alterations of vision caused by macular degeneration.

Macular degeneration also needs to be differentiated from two other common eye conditions that affect many elderly people: cataracts and glaucoma.

A cataract is a clouding of the lens of the eye. Situated just behind the pupil, the lens is normally crystal clear and focuses, or refracts, light rays onto the retina, which is the light-sensitive layer at the rear of the eye. (The anatomy of the eye is covered in more detail in chapter 4.) There are many types of cataracts, usually described by the location of the hazy spots within the lens. As light enters the pupil it can be partially blocked or bent by the hazy spots in the lens, resulting in an overall haziness of vision. This is often described by the patient as seeing through a fog or veil, with a general, uniform decrease in the sharpness of images. This differs significantly from the altered vision of macular degeneration, which is distorted or blurred but only in the central area of your field of focus.

Glaucoma is a fairly common eye disease; it usually causes no symptoms until moderately advanced. This condition, associated with an increased pressure of the fluid within the eyeball, causes gradual damage to the optic nerve, resulting in a loss of visual function that is quite different from that of macular degeneration.

Glaucoma causes a slow deterioration in peripheral, or side, vision—just the opposite of macular degeneration. Here's a good way to visualize the difference between glaucoma and macular degeneration. Someone who has advanced glaucoma sees the world as if he or she is looking through a narrow pipe, like a gun barrel. Someone with severe macular degeneration, on the other hand, would look at a person's face and see only the hair, ears, and chin.

Cataracts are treated very successfully with surgery, in which the lens is removed and replaced by a plastic lens. Glaucoma, if diagnosed early, can be treated with medicines to prevent vision loss. Unfortunately, solutions are not so easily obtained with macular degeneration.

No Pattern of Vision Loss

Another difference between visual changes associated with macular degeneration and those caused by other conditions is the nature of the progression. With cataracts, for instance, visual loss is gradual and becomes apparent mostly when measured in the doctor's office. With macular degeneration, however, there is no set pattern of vision loss. In many people, vision may remain stable for years, while in others, a significant decrease in vision may occur overnight. With most patients, the visual changes seem to occur over a short period of time and then level off until other changes take place, again over a short period. However, some macular degeneration patients, those who have what's called the "wet" form of the disease, may suffer an abrupt and marked decrease in vision. (The different types of macular degeneration will be discussed in chapter 4.)

At some point, though, vision loss for most macular degeneration patients progresses to the point where one's lifestyle has to change. Driving may become impossible. Reading becomes difficult, routine tasks become sources of frustration, and television is no longer as enjoyable as it once was. Remember, there are ways to surmount these obstacles. You will never be blind. You will never need to be guided by the arm or told where to sit or to be careful of your head. You will be able to read and write, converse with friends, and listen to music you love. You will still be able to function as a loving father, mother, grandfather, grandmother, sister, brother, or friend. Your life will continue to be as fulfilled and as joyous as you care to make it. In short, life will continue to have many rewards, and with some effort, almost all vision-related impairments can be overcome.

CHAPTER 3

Understanding Your Vision

Readers of a certain age may well remember the common folk wisdom that if you have weak eyes, you should save your sight by using them sparingly. Amazingly, this view was still widely held until about the middle of the twentieth century. Wrongheaded acceptance of this nonsense was indicative of simplistic thinking about sight even among health care professionals, who until about the 1950s divided eye patients into one of two categories: sighted or blind. Patients were either given the best possible glasses or taught Braille.

The awareness that visual disability could be partial really arose after World War II, when many service-related eye injuries were treated in ways that enabled the veterans to gain employment. Low-vision aids were prescribed and a basic definition of low vision evolved. That definition of low vision relates to the way eyesight is measured.

Defining Vision in Terms of Function

Before discussing how vision is measured and low vision defined, let me say that I believe, along with many low-vision specialists, that the best way to define low vision is in terms of function—what a person can and can't do when his or her vision is corrected by the best possible eyeglasses. For example, a fifty-year-old truck driver who with the strongest possible eyeglasses has 20/60 vision is considered to have low vision, since he can no longer function in his job. On the other hand, consider a macular degeneration patient such as my eighty-four-year-old aunt, who lives in an assisted living center. She enjoys watching television and reads all she likes by removing her glasses, which correct her severe nearsightedness. Her uncorrected nearsighted, or myopic, vision allows her to read by holding papers very close to her eyes. Functionally, she needs no low-vision correction.

To help you better understand your vision and to dispel fears about being legally blind, let me explain the two key measurements of vision: visual acuity and visual field.

Visual Acuity: The Eye-Chart Measurement

Visual acuity is measured in the 20/20-style notation, which is commonly spoken of but rarely well understood. Visual acuity refers to the clarity of a row of letters or symbols that a person can see compared with what a theoretical "normal-sighted" person could see at the same distance. Visual acuity is measured with the familiar eye chart, made up of rows of different-sized letters. When an eye doctor measures your visual acuity, you are stationed twenty feet away from the chart (the distance is typically simulated in a doctor's office by adjusting the size of the letters) and you identify the smallest row of letters that you can see clearly. The result is compared with a standard of so-called normal vision. If the smallest row of letters that you can read from twenty feet could be read by a normal-sighted person from sixty feet, your uncorrected visual acuity would be stated as 20/60.

Of course, most people don't have natural 20/20 vision. They need glasses to correct their visual acuity to 20/20, or as close to it as possible in each eye. Remember that the only meaningful visual measurement is your visual acuity with glasses. If your uncorrected vision is 20/80, but with glasses your visual acuity is 20/20, you do not have a visual impairment. People are considered to have low vision only if the visual acuity in their better-seeing eye is 20/50 or worse with the best correction they can get from eyeglasses.

Visual Field: Side Vision

The second measure of vision is called visual field. This is a measurement of so-called peripheral, or side, vision. Each eye, tested separately while staring at a point directly ahead, can still see objects to the right and left and above and below eye level. The visual fields of each eye overlap, but not completely. Each eye can see roughly in a semicircle of 180 degrees to the sides, or horizontally, and somewhat less in the vertical direction. Certain diseases like glaucoma shrink the size of the field of vision to 60 degrees, 40 degrees, or even less. On the other hand, macular degeneration does not affect peripheral vision at all, but—as we've discussed—creates a blurry, distorted, or even opaque "island" of vision loss in the general center of the visual field.

A final note now on what it means to be legally blind, and what it doesn't mean. Measurements of visual acuity and visual field both play a role in the definition of legal blindness, a concept that evolved in the 1930s to determine who would be entitled to government assistance because of visual impairment. The definition that evolved for legal blindness was set as having either a visual acuity of 20/200 in the better eye with the best possible eyeglasses, or a visual field of less than 20 degrees in the better eye, even if the visual acuity in that eye is normal. If you are legally blind it means that you are eligible for certain government benefits, such as an additional exemption on your tax return. But being legally blind does not mean that you can't see. In fact, most people classified as legally blind have considerable useful vision.

At some point in the course of our disease, most people with macular degeneration will become classified as having low vision. Many of us—but certainly not most—will be further classified as legally blind. But before we turn to a discussion of how to cope with low vision, let's spend some time developing a better understanding of macular degeneration.

CHAPTER 4

What Exactly Is Macular Degeneration?

The eye is a truly wondrous organ. The ever-changing complexity of images that it presents to us, the incredible depth of three-dimensionality, the ability to discern minute differences in hues of all colors, the capacity to rapidly change focus and track objects, and the seeding of vivid visual details or panoramas into our memory banks—all these are just some of the wonderful capacities of the eye.

The remarkable importance of the eye to survival is indicated by the fact that of the twelve vital cranial nerves from the brain, six are totally concerned with the function of the eye. The remaining six are concerned with everything else—such activities as hearing, smelling, tasting, breathing, and maintaining the heartbeat. It is as if our Maker recognized the great importance of vision and its intrinsic complexity and dedicated fully half of the most vital controlling nerves of our entire body to our eyes.

The complexity of the eye is manifested most dramatically by the incredible rapidity with which images change in the brain. This can be demonstrated simply by moving your gaze quickly from point to point around a room. The image of the clock in that room is instantaneously replaced by that of a chair, a calendar, a pencil, or a book. When we pause to consider that the images we see are also in full color and are constantly moving, we begin to appreciate the fantastic complexity of vision.

The Anatomy of the Eye

To better understand the changes in vision that occur with macular degeneration, we must first have some notion of the anatomy of this amazing organ and the process of sight. Think of the eyeball as a sphere somewhat smaller than a Ping-Pong ball. Imagine a half-inch-round opening cut out of one side, the front. Opposite that would be an eighth-inch-thick cord extending out from behind the sphere.

The opening in front is covered with a clear plastic disc bulging slightly outward, the cornea. Think of the optic nerve as the cord running along the side of the head to end at the rear of the brain.

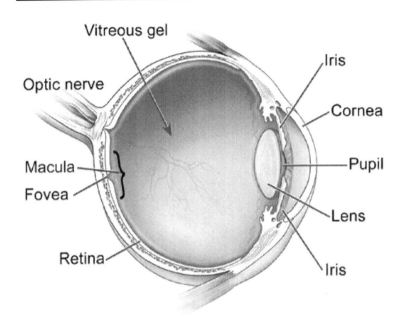

National Eye Institute

An eighth of an inch behind our cornea is a half-inch-diameter "curtain," the blue or brownish iris with a hole in its center. The iris is composed of a very thin muscle layer that enlarges or reduces the size of the central hole, which is called the pupil.

Directly behind the iris is the lens of the eye. This is a slightly flattened pea-shaped object, crystal clear and suspended directly behind the pupil by fine fibers radiating outward toward the spherical white shell of our eyeball, called the sclera. Lining the very inside of the eye is the delicate transparent retina, composed of over a million nerve cells and their supporting tissue. If you then imagine all the fibers from these retinal nerve cells joining together to form the optic nerve, you will have a good three-dimensional image of the eye.

How We See

Now we know what the eye looks like, but how do we see?

Seeing basically involves light. When we gaze at an object, we are really seeing its image as reflected by the light bouncing off it. The light waves enter the eye through the cornea, which serves not only to protect the eye but also to focus the light through the pupil. The iris's job is to adjust the size of the pupil, enlarging it in dim light to help us see better and constricting it in bright light to protect the sensitive retina. After passing through the pupil, the light waves reach the lens, which refocuses them with pinpoint precision onto the retina. If we think of the eye's lens as akin to the lens of a traditional camera, the retina would be analogous to the camera's film. The retina consists of millions of light-sensitive nerve cells, called rods and cones, that capture the image of the object being regarded. The image is then conveyed through the optic nerve to the brain, where it is interpreted, recorded, and acted upon.

The Role of the Retina

Let us focus our attention for a moment on the retina, for that is the part of the eye with which you will be most concerned. All parts of the retina contribute to seeing, but the most important part is a small circular area about the size of a pinhead, the macula. This tiny island of tissue is responsible for what we all regard as the most important function of our vision: the ability to focus directly on small, specific objects. This involves reading, detailed discrimination of faces and form, appreciation of color with its full intensity, and the ability to finely track movement with depth perception.

If the macula becomes damaged from a degenerative process, we lose some or all of our central, detailed vision. The term *macular degeneration* applies to various diseases that lead to the deterioration of the macula.

Our concern, of course, is age-related macular degeneration, which is the leading cause of visual impairment in people over fifty years of age in the United States. The physiological mechanisms of age-related macular degeneration are detailed at the end of this chapter in a section for the technically curious. But the key thing for everyone to appreciate is that once the delicate, light-sensing nerve cells of the macula are damaged or destroyed, they cannot be repaired or regenerated. They and their function are lost forever. When many cells in the macula become damaged, our central vision becomes obscured by a perpetually cloudy spot called a scotoma. This central scotoma, which is always with us, makes it maddeningly difficult for those of us with macular degeneration to read, recognize faces, and otherwise live the lives we were used to.

"Dry" Versus "Wet" AMD

There are two forms of age-related macular degeneration. The more common form—and fortunately the less severe of the two—is referred to as the dry type. The dry type of AMD evolves slowly, first in one eye and then usually in the other. It is marked by a thinning of the light-sensing cells in the macula, as increasing numbers of these cells are destroyed due to the still-unexplained degenerative process. This process typically occurs over a matter of years, and its progression may be faster at some times than others. With many people, the degenerative process simply stops before vision loss becomes severe.

The second type of age-related macular degeneration is called the wet type, or more technically, the neovascular or exudative form of the disease. While far less common than the dry type, the wet type leads to a far greater visual impairment. In wet AMD, new, abnormal blood vessels begin growing under the macula. Leaking blood and fluid from these vessels can quickly kill the sensitive cells of the macula, leading to a rather dramatic loss of vision within a period of weeks or months.

The Significance of Drusen

Drusen are the early warning signs of both types of age-related macular degeneration. These are tiny yellowish deposits of waste material that accumulate in the retina. In younger eyes, the waste material is removed and recycled quite effectively, but the process doesn't work so well in the elderly. Fortunately, most drusen are simply benign signs of aging. It takes a careful examination by an ophthalmologist, however, to determine whether drusen are benign or are possible predictors of future trouble. Drusen are visible with an ophthalmoscope. They are not visible externally, nor to an untrained examiner, since they can be very tiny.

Depending on their nature, size, and location, some drusen can weaken the delicate tissue of the retina enough to allow small blood vessels to grow in areas where they don't belong, specifically under the macula. If those "rogue" blood vessels leak blood or fluid under the macula, it would lead to the wet form of AMD.

The role of drusen is less understood in the more common dry type of age-related macular degeneration. However, the presence of drusen is so prevalent among patients with dry AMD that it is considered a defining characteristic of the disease. At this point you may be wondering, "If I have the low-risk, dry AMD, what are the chances that I will get the more dangerous wet AMD?" Fortunately, those chances are very small; for most people with dry AMD there is about a 1 percent chance of developing the wet type within five years. However, if the drusen begin enlarging or otherwise changing shape, the risk can increase to as high as a 10 percent chance of developing wet AMD within five years.

Why You Should Monitor Your AMD

As mentioned earlier, only an examination by an ophthalmologist can determine if the drusen in a retina are benign or are the precursor to wet AMD. If the latter, further tests can identify any rogue blood vessels, which are the causal agent of wet AMD. With new laser treatments (see chapter 6), your doctor may be able to destroy these abnormal blood vessels before they leak and damage the macula.

I'd like to emphasize two points about laser treatments. First, laser treatment is applicable only to wet AMD; it can do nothing for the more prevalent dry type of the disease. And second, laser treatment can't reverse existing damage to the macula; its only use is to possibly prevent further damage.

Everyone with age-related macular degeneration must keep up with their scheduled visits to the ophthalmologist because the sooner your doctor can detect signs of rogue blood vessels, the better the chances of treating them.

When you were diagnosed with age-related macular degeneration, your eye doctor probably gave you a self-test card called an Amsler grid. This is simply a card with a grid of intersecting horizontal and vertical lines and a dot at the center. If, when you look at the dot, some of the lines appear wavy or are not visible at all, it could be a sign that rogue blood vessels are forming and you should consult your ophthalmologist immediately. To help detect signs of wet AMD at the earliest possible time, you should conduct this self-test regularly—preferably weekly, but no less frequently than every month. (If you've lost your Amsler grid, you can use the one printed in the back of this book.)

Now that we have a better understanding of macular degeneration, we can move on to a discussion of the possible causes of the disease. Those readers who would like a more detailed discussion of eyesight and the anatomy of the retina may wish first to review the following section.

Visual Tracking and Accommodation

"Tracking" and "accommodation" play important roles in our vision. Tracking refers to the need for the two eyes to coordinate so precisely and move together so exactly that the light coming from even the smallest object is focused on the retina of each eye at precisely the same instant. If this does not occur, the brain will be presented with two views of the same object and will be very confused.

The manner in which the eyes move simultaneously and equally in all directions is accomplished by the six muscle strips attached to each eye. These muscles are activated by nerves from the brain that respond to light entering the eye or sound from the ear. The reflexive, as opposed to voluntary, movement of the eyes allows us the protection of a radar-like system to sound and light. There is, of course, also the conscious movement of the eyes that we all do in following any object of interest.

The process called accommodation can be best likened to the autofocus technology in many modern cameras. When the light from an object reaches the retina, an immediate message is sent along the nerves to the brain and then back along other nerves to the ciliary muscle of the eye. This very thin muscle lines a quarter-inch strip of the inside of the scleral wall in the shape of a ring surrounding the site of the lens of the eye. It appears as a halo of muscle attached to the lens by fine fibers radiating from the muscle to the lens.

When the nerve message from the brain tells this muscle that the retinal image is not in exact focus, the muscle either contracts or relaxes and thus changes the shape of the lens. This occurs to the exact degree needed to focus light from an object at any distance clearly upon the retina. This action is of particular importance for bringing into focus objects that are one to two feet from the eye, such as reading material.

Difficulty in reading is experienced by almost everyone over age forty-five, since the elasticity of the lens, and therefore its ability to change focus, rapidly diminishes from that age. This results in the need for the focusing power of reading glasses.

Retinal Anatomy and Physiology

The retina is less than tissue paper thin, transparent, and composed of two basic layers. The innermost layer, lying in contact with the vitreous gel, is the neurosensory retina—the cells that receive and process the light energy. The outer layer of the retina is called the retinal pigment epithelium, known to all eye specialists as the RPE.

The neurosensory layer of the retina itself has ten distinct layers, in contrast to the single layer of cells in the RPE. These multiple layers consist primarily of the nuclei of cells in the visual pathway and their axons, or nerve fibers. These fibers, in turn, converge within the retina toward the back of the eye, where they join together to form the million fibers of the optic nerve.

The placement of each layer in this exquisitely thin membrane, the retina, is brilliant. Consider that the most important cells in the process of seeing are the rods and cones. In a photographic film, for example, the sensitive layer is that which is struck first by light. In the retina, the layer of light-sensing cells called rods and cones require so much energy to convert light to image that they must be in direct contact with the body's energy source, our blood. Consequently, the rod and cone layer is the rearmost layer of the retina, lying next to the RPE (retinal pigment epithelium). Light must therefore pass through all the other cellular and support layers of the retina before it reaches the light-sensitive zone.

There are many more rods than cones in the retina. Rods extend from the very edge of the retina near the front of the eye to all but the central part of the macula at the back of the eye. This central macula, or fovea, is composed solely of cones and has no overlying layers like the rest of the retina. This ingenious arrangement allows the macula's cones to receive light unobstructed by retinal nerve fiber layers and thus gain even more acuity.

There are roughly 150 million rods to 10 million cones in each eye. If you place a rod in a microscope, you will see a cylinder connected to a small spherical nucleus that extends an axon to the next layer of connecting cells, the bipolar cells. The cylindrical part of the rod is the light-transmitting factory. This rod outer segment, or ROS, is gently covered and almost enveloped by darkly pigmented fingers of tissue extending from the overlying cells of the RPE.

The function of these enveloping "fingers" is to act like a darkroom around each cone to prevent the scatter from the light rays, which would blur the activities of the adjacent rods. The cylinder is made up of a protein called opsin, which is in a continual process of joining up with a derivative of vitamin A called retinol in one part of the cylinder while breaking away from it in another part.

The joining together of retinol and opsin forms rhodopsin, (formerly called visual purple), while the breaking apart occurs when triggered by the energy impact of even the tiniest amount of light, called a photon. The breakup of the molecule of rhodopsin results in a sudden actual elongation of its molecular structure (a process called isomerization), which changes the static electrical charge on the cell membrane of the rod. This minute change in cellular electrical charge is transmitted to the bipolar cells, which transmit it to the ganglion cells and thence all the way to the brain.

The vital rhodopsin in the cylinder part of our rod cell is layered in the cylinder like the coins in a roll of nickels. As the visual process continues, the "coins" are moved, as they break down, toward the retinal pigment epithelium cells, which essentially "digest" these tips as they are shed. The RPE cells then replenish more retinol from vitamin A to the rods in order to form more rhodopsin. The RPE cells also discharge the broken-down vitamin A and the remnants of opsin into the bloodstream of the choroid, which is the vascular layer lying between the retina and the sclera. The RPE then takes from the choroidal blood fresh vitamin A and amino acids to re-form the entire rhodopsin molecule.

The layered-coin formation of rhodopsin in the rod cylinder is an inspired way to gain the maximum exposure of rhodopsin to light. Even a small amount of light will trigger a large breakdown of this protein molecule to generate an electrical impulse, thus transmitting light-electrical conduction.

I have concentrated on the function of a rod for two reasons. First, rod vision chemistry has been studied extensively. Second, cones behave in a similar fashion but have a more complex protein structure, since there are three types of cones. There are separate cones for red, blue, and green color reception. These blend in a delicate manner to transmit the wavelength of any of the hundreds of different hues that our brain can discern.

The brain, after all, is the organ responsible for vision. The exact location of the vision center is in the occipital lobe at the back of the head. This is where all the electrical impulses, starting from the rods and cones, going from the bipolar cells to the ganglion cells on a long course along both outer sides of the brain, end in the cells of the visual cortex in the occipital lobe. The fact that it is our brain that "sees" is proven when a severe injury occurs to the back of the brain, following which a person may become totally blind while having eyes that function normally.

For our story, the most vital portion of the retina is the circular area of retinal tissue about an eighth of an inch in diameter that lies about a quarter of an inch to the right of the right optic nerve and a quarter of an inch to the left of the left optic nerve. This area can be thought of as a target of several concentric rings. The bull's-eye is the fovea, composed only of cones and with no overlying cells or nerve fibers. Each of the cones in the fovea connects with one ganglion cell going directly to the brain. In other parts of the retina, each cone or rod connects to many ganglion cells, decreasing its effective output to the brain.

The outlying circles of the target contain decreasing numbers of cones and increasing numbers of rods. This is very important for people with fovea problems because if the cones just outside the fovea are intact, vision can still be as good as 20/40. If, however, only the edge of the macula circle is intact, there are only enough cones to yield approximately 20/200 vision.

Our cones are the key to clear, sharp, full-color vision. The rods provide us with the ability to see forms in dimmer light, but even with no macula cone function a person's vision should not deteriorate below 20/300. This is the scientific basis for assuring AMD patients that they will certainly never be blind.

Diagnostic Tools

Current diagnosis and treatment of AMD requires careful photography of the retina and especially of the macula to search out early signs of degeneration. The typical angiogram is a rapid sequence of photographs of the retina. A fluorescent dye is injected into a vein in the forearm, and then a series of pictures are taken through the pupil while the dye courses through the vessels of the retina.

The photos show up abnormalities as defects in the normal circulatory pattern. Digital photography, now available for standard cameras as well, creates computer images that can be manipulated, stored, and transmitted; such photography will allow the retinologist to finely hone his or her diagnostic ability and laser treatment skills.

Fluorescein angiography has been the gold standard of retinal diagnosis since it was first introduced in 1961. It provides information about the retina, the choroidal circulation, the status of the retinal pigment epithelium (RPE), and the presence or absence of subretinal fluid or hemorrhage. Although it is very valuable, it is not indicated for every patient or on every visit. New developments will improve its ability to diagnose AMD and many other retinal abnormalities.

Indocyanine green angiography is a form of digital photography of the retina utilizing a dye called indocyanine green (ICG), which is injected into a vein in the arm. Unlike the fluorescein dye of fluorescein angiography, ICG reveals more details of the choroidal circulation in addition to the retinal circulation. This allows detection of what is called occult choroidal neovascularization. *Occult* simply refers to the fact that these small new blood vessel buds were not visible with standard fluorescein angiography. By making them visible with ICG, these vessel tufts may be treated earlier and more effectively.

A new diagnostic imaging technique called optical coherence tomography, or OCT, produces detailed images of the retina and macula as if they were sliced by a knife and looked at in cross section—that is to say, the view is of the cut edge. It is similar to an MRI or a CT scan; the former uses magnetic resonance and the latter, x-rays. In OCT, light waves are used, and with no patient discomfort. In many cases great detail can be observed. New blood vessels forming under the macula may be invisible to the usual angiogram or photographs of the macula but will show up distinctly with OCT. This, of course, could also lead to earlier treatment before these occult blood vessels could bleed.

CHAPTER 5

What Causes Age-Related Macular Degeneration?

After "Will I go blind?" the most frequently asked question by new macular degeneration patients is usually "Why did I get this disease?" While we have a definitive answer for the first question *(no!)*, we do not have a satisfactory answer for the second.

Essentially, we don't know what causes macular degeneration. What we do know is this: age-related macular degeneration is not caused by a bacteria, a virus, or a fungus. It is not caused by a tumor, cancer, or injury. It is certainly not contagious. And it may affect one eye later than the other not by somehow spreading from one eye to the other, but rather by a time delay in the basic, as yet unknown causative process.

One reason so little is known about the cause of age-related macular degeneration is that, compared with other major causes of vision loss, it represents a relatively new area of study for ophthalmologists. The first actual mention of the treatment of eye diseases probably dates back to ancient Egyptian writings of nearly five thousand years ago, where there is mention of a heavy mascara-like pigment being applied around the eyelids and having a protective effect against what was probably the disease known today as trachoma, a highly contagious disease of the eyelids and cornea. We also see a reference to the study of eye disease in the Code of Hammurabi, the Babylonian king of about 2200 BCE, where there is a description of the treatment of diseases of the tear sac, which lies at the inner corner of the lower eyelid.

Of the two major blinding diseases, cataracts and glaucoma, the former has been known for hundreds of years, but it was not until the early twentieth century that a reliable surgical procedure for treating cataracts was developed. And it wasn't until the middle of the nineteenth century that doctors developed a full understanding of glaucoma.

Now fast-forward another hundred years, to the mid-twentieth century, and take a look at the ophthalmology texts then being used by young medical students like me. You would find that age-related macular degeneration, the eye disease that now causes more visual impairment in the industrialized world than any other, was barely noted in those textbooks. This does not mean that it did not exist at that time, but only that the means to detect it and the desire to study it were lacking.

In fact, it wasn't until the 1960s—over a hundred years after the invention of the ophthalmoscope allowed doctors to look at a living human retina—that ophthalmologists were finally able to fully analyze the effects of macular degeneration.

The breakthrough came with the development of fluorescein angiography in 1961. This procedure, which allows ophthalmologists to see extraordinary levels of detail in the retina and macula, may have been used to help diagnose your case of macular degeneration. It involves the injection of a safe dye into the vein of an arm. The dye reaches the blood vessels of the retina, and when an eye doctor uses an ophthalmoscope to shine a blue light in the eye, the dye fluoresces, or glows, and thus outlines any abnormalities in the blood vessels. It would also indicate whether blood or fluid has leaked into the surrounding tissues. The images can be captured on film with a special camera affixed to a biomicroscope, or slit lamp. The camera is designed to take pictures rapidly—every few seconds—to follow the course of the dye through the retinal arteries and veins, thereby outlining any disturbance in the anatomy of the macula.

Before fluorescein angiography, careful delineation of the various forms of macular degeneration was not possible. Indeed, it was impossible to even discuss the causes of many other common retinal conditions and most macular problems. (No one really knew, for example, what caused President Theodore Roosevelt to suddenly lose the vision in his left eye after a boxing match in the early 1900s, although today we can surmise that he remained blind in that eye because of a retinal detachment.)

Unfortunately, with all the detailed knowledge we now have of the anatomy of diseased maculas and the specifics of functional vision loss, even down to a cellular level, we have few conclusions about the real cause of macular degeneration. This is enormously frustrating for eye doctors (not to mention AMD patients), because much is known about the causes of other types of macular disease. For instance, some forms of macular disease may be caused by a fungus, as in ocular histoplasmosis, a disease found most often in the Mississippi and Ohio River valleys. A form of macular degeneration can also be caused by a particular parasite carried by cats and passed to humans, a condition known as toxoplasmosis. The virus of rubella (German measles) can also cause macular damage in children, while in adults CMV (cytomegalovirus) may result in macular damage.

Even though we are not sure about what causes age-related macular degeneration, we do have some theories. It appears likely that AMD may be caused, at least in part, by one or more of the following factors:

- The normal aging process
- Heredity

- Toxins such as tobacco smoke, alcohol, and certain medications

- Environmental factors, such as exposure to ultraviolet light

- Nutritional issues, such as a lack of certain vitamins, minerals, or plant chemicals

- Being overweight

Normal Aging

The most obvious possible cause of age-related macular degeneration is the aging process itself. As we get older, the human body just doesn't work as well as it did when we were younger. Our metabolism changes. Injuries may take longer to heal. Our eyes are particularly susceptible to age-related changes. After age forty, most people need reading glasses, and the likelihood of developing cataracts rises significantly after age sixty. So perhaps the eye's ability to maintain a healthy retina also suffers with age, leading to the degeneration of the macula.

The association between aging and retinal deterioration has been confirmed by many studies of the microscopic appearance of the retina at different ages in people with normal eyes. Many age-related changes cannot be seen with any method of examination in a healthy living eye, but instead have been observed microscopically in post mortem specimens. There is, for example, a general reduction in the density and distribution of rods and cones, the retinal cells that are responsible for light reception.

But not everyone over age seventy gets macular degeneration, so there are probably other factors at work. Here is a look at the most likely culprits.

Heredity

There is growing evidence that heredity plays a significant role in age-related macular degeneration. Certain people may be predisposed to developing macular degeneration later in life because of a genetic malfunction. Researchers are beginning to suspect that an as-yet-unidentified defective gene may interfere with the eye's ability to "digest" the microscopic bits of waste material that are constantly being shed in the process of seeing. The buildup of this waste material, which in normal eyes is "recycled," leads to the creation of drusen, which in turn may form the basis for degenerative changes in the macula, as discussed earlier.

But what causes this genetic malfunction? We don't know. Perhaps it is a hereditary problem, in which the gene is programmed to malfunction late in life. Or perhaps, again because of heredity, the gene that directs the recycling of the eye's waste material is susceptible to damage by environmental factors, toxins, or nutritional deficiencies. For additional, very recent findings in the genetics of AMD, please read the last segment of this chapter entitled "Genetic Biology."

Smoking

Smoking has its primary deadly effect on the heart and lungs, where it causes a general reduction in blood oxygen levels. Reduced oxygen levels are a particular hazard for the eye because, for its size, the eye needs more oxygen than any other organ in the body. If you exclude the vitreous humor that fills the eyeball, the eye is only about one-sixtieth the size of the heart, yet it consumes sixty times as much oxygen as the heart. Moreover, nicotine causes a narrowing of the eye's blood vessels, and it also has a direct effect on the ganglian, or nerve cells, in the retina. The link between smoking and age-related macular degeneration has been supported by several studies. These studies indicate that smokers have double the risk of developing AMD, and that the risk increases with the number of cigarettes smoked daily.

Alcohol

Whether alcohol has an effect on the eye, especially

the macula, is still inconclusive. We know that alcohol in substantial amounts can act like tobacco in having a toxic effect on the nerve cells of the retina. However, there are studies that appear to demonstrate that wine (but not beer or spirits) may actually be beneficial in preventing age-related macular degeneration. One study indicated that consuming one to four glasses of wine a month seems to be statistically helpful. It would seem prudent with alcohol use to limit your intake to a single drink a day.

Medications

The possibility that a drug or medication may have a specific adverse effect on the macula does exist. One medication, chloroquin, an agent commonly used in the treatment of lupus and some forms of arthritis, can cause a specific form of macular degeneration. Fortunately, if the early signs of this toxicity are observed by an eye specialist, the condition is reversible if the drug is discontinued. Anyone taking this medication should be carefully examined by an ophthalmologist about every six months.

Although they are no longer commonly used, two medications for psychiatric disorders, Mellaril and Thorazine, can cause a specific type of change in the macula with the prolonged use of high doses. A more commonly used medication, digitalis, can occasionally cause a dysfunction of the eye's cones, resulting in a peculiar yellowish vision. Fortunately, this is also reversible with cessation or reduction of drug dosage. Tamoxifen, a drug used with success in the treatment of breast cancer, may lead to shiny little deposits in the macula with some loss of central vision, but this is also, fortunately, rare.

Environmental Factors

Air pollutants—primarily particulate matter, sulfur dioxide, carbon monoxide, and nitrogen oxides—have a negative effect on the human cardiovascular and respiratory systems, and consequently may contribute to visual problems. For instance, there is a known link between carbon monoxide and visual perceptive loss. Other pollutants can have an indirect effect on the eye.

The growing problem with the earth's ozone layer also may be a factor in the evident increase in certain eye diseases such as cataracts and AMD. Since 1974, scientists have observed a depletion of the earth's protective ozone layer, due in large part to the use of chlorofluorocarbons, which are chemicals used in refrigerants, air conditioning, packaging, and aerosol propellants. What all this has to do with vision relates to the damage that we know ultraviolet light does to the lens of the eye, and to a lesser degree to the macula.

As the ozone layer continues to thin out due to natural and man-made causes, it becomes ever more important to protect your eyes from the damaging effects of these ultraviolet rays. In other words, people with macular degeneration or early cataracts should always wear sunglasses adequate to protect their eyes from ultraviolet light.

With all that I have said about how damaging ultraviolet rays can be, you might think studies have definitely implicated excessive sunlight as a cause of age-related macular degeneration. Although we are aware of the damaging effect of ultraviolet light on the lens of the eye, as in cataract formation, the relationship of ultraviolet light to age-related macular degeneration is less clear, though it is highly suggestive. The ability of visible blue light to affect rods and cones has been noted. For this reason, everyone should wear UV-absorbing glasses whenever exposed to sunlight. This should cut down on the incidence of cataract formation and will probably be beneficial to the macula as well.

Nutrition

Certain nutrients are vital to the health of the eye, and chapter 7 concerns the role of nutrition in age-related macular degeneration. For now, though, it is important to understand that a diet deficient in certain essential nutrients could be involved in the development of age-related macular degeneration. The most important substance is a nutrient called lutein, which is found most plentifully in leafy green vegetables such as spinach, kale, and collard greens. Studies published in prestigious journals such as the *Journal of the American Medical Association,* the *British Medical Journal,* the *American Journal of Nutrition,* and *Investigative Ophthalmology* all support the belief that there is a relationship between a diet rich in lutein and a lower incidence of macular degeneration and cataract formation.

Now what is this lutein, which most people have never heard of? Lutein and its very close relative zeaxanthin are carotinoids, part of a group of red and yellow pigment chemicals that are found in high concentration in green leafy vegetables and also in other fruits and vegetables. Lutein is known to be an important antioxidant. Lutein and zeaxanthin are also the only two phyto-chemicals (chemicals found in plants) found in the eye, and they are essential to the eye's health. They are primarily located in the macula, and to a lesser degree in the lens of the eye.

The normal amount of lutein in the lens of the eye usually helps protect the clear lens fibers from becoming cloudy and forming a cataract. The lutein in the macula may protect the light-sensitive rods and cones. It probably does this in two ways. First, it prevents harmful free radicals from interacting with the rich lipid layer in the retina, thereby reducing the amount of fatty substance that may cause more drusen. (Drusen, as discussed earlier, are the waste buildups often associated with macular degeneration.) Secondly, the yellowish color of the lutein may actually absorb more of the bluish light that strikes the retina and which may cause more photooxidative (light-induced) damage to the delicate macula cells.

Body Weight and General Health

The body mass index, or BMI, is the measurement of the relative percentages of fat and muscle mass in the human body. A person's BMI appears to be directly linked to his or her likelihood of developing age-related macular degeneration. Studies have shown a definite increase in instances of age-related macular degeneration among individuals, particularly men, with a BMI greater than 27, which would be associated with being moderately to significantly overweight.

Other general health risk factors, such as diabetes, hypertension, arterial sclerosis, and cardiac disease, have not been definitely implicated in the development of age-related macular degeneration. However, it is only prudent to maintain optimal control of any of these conditions to avoid any degree of damage to the circulatory, hormonal, or nutritional well-being of the macula and the rest of the retina—indeed, the entire eye.

A New Theory

The very recent development of laser Doppler flow measurements, the ability to measure the actual amount of blood flowing in the blood vessels behind the retina, has provided fascinating information about retinal function. Apparently, the blood flow behind the macula that nourishes it may begin to diminish as the first sign of the disease. The decreased flow may then cause the whole chain of degeneration.

This fascinating theory of the cause of age-related macular degeneration is based on the actual finding of decreased blood flow in the vessels behind the retina. According to this theory, AMD may be *due* to the decreased flow rather than the *cause* of the decreased flow. The diminished blood flow, in turn, may be due to the "stiffening" of the delicate tissues within the eye. This stiffening may be due to age and deficiencies in diet. Although this theory is speculative at present, it does open up an entirely new area of research that may help all patients with macular degeneration.

The Bottom Line

So what does all this mean to the patient with age-related macular degeneration? Clearly, if you are reading this book you probably already have the condition (or are connected to someone who does) so it is too late to prevent it by avoiding known risk factors. Perhaps you are one of the many people with age-related macular degeneration who have always taken good care of themselves. The fact of the matter is that we really do not know with certainty why anyone gets macular degeneration. But while the effects of macular degeneration can't be reversed, it seems possible—indeed, even likely—that they can be slowed by following a lifestyle that in any case will do no harm and will almost certainly lead to other health benefits:

- Don't smoke.

- Drink moderately.

- Eat lots of vegetables, especially spinach.

- Always use high-quality sunglasses when you're outside.

- Don't gain weight.

Aging and the Retina

There have been many studies of the microscopic appearance of the retina, the RPE, and the choroid at different ages in people with normal eyes. With aging, in addition to a general reduction in the density and distribution of rods and cones, the pigment epithelium (RPE) loses granules of pigment and the number of drusen increase. Drusen are also found in Bruch's membrane, which lies between the RPE and the choroid. The choroidal layer of fine blood vessels also shows signs of arterial sclerotic change (hardening of the blood vessel wall) and often some new blood vessel formation (neovascularization) beginning to form in the cracks of Bruch's membrane.

Genetic Biology

With the exception of the sperm or ovum, every cell in your body, all 100 trillion of them, contains forty-six chromosomes, or twenty-three from your mother and twenty-three matching ones from your father. Each chromosome, looking like a tiny piece of irregular ribbon, consists of a very long chemical macromolecule called DNA (deoxyribonucleic acid). This molecule is a complex grouping of five atoms: carbon, oxygen, hydrogen, nitrogen and phosphorous. The intricate arrangement of billions of these atoms into six smaller molecules, billions of which form an actual ladder-like arrangement, the macromolecule DNA. This very long molecule in the chromosome is twisted to form the famous "Double Helix" form discovered by Watson and Crick in 1953. These strands of DNA are then coiled like spaghetti to form each of the differently shaped 23 pairs of chromosomes, which are in every cell nucleus. To gain some idea of the enormous complexity of DNA, think of this structure as the long strands of spaghetti coiled tightly in each of the 46 chromosomes in each cell nucleus. Experiments have shown that if one could "unravel" and splice together all the strands of DNA in one cell, it would reach six feet in length! If you then, in theory, could tie together such strands from each of the 100 trillion cells in your body, the resulting theoretical "string" would stretch how far? Across the country? No. Around the earth? No. Actually 100 times to the sun and back!

Which brings us back to consider the roughly 100,000 genes, which are within the coiled DNA Helix in each of the 46 chromosomes in each and every cell of your body. A gene is simply a section, sometimes short, sometimes very long, of the DNA strand in a particular chromosome. The gene consists of a variable length of the "sides of the ladder" (sugars plus phosphates) together with a variable number of "rungs of the ladder" (some combination of the "bases" A, T, C, G (adenine, thymine, cytosine or guanine). A gene may be composed of just a few of such segments or up to hundreds of them.

At present, science knows the function of only a small number of genes, perhaps eight thousand of them. But we are going to focus on only one of them as a primary suspect in the overall genetic basis of macular degeneration.

Geneticists have determined the location of certain genes which control specific functions or structures within the body and the diseases which occur when some of the A, T, C or G are different or missing,(called a mutation). These mutations can occur naturally or be inherited. It is in one tiny spot of chromosome number one called 1Q32 that a mutation has been found to be common in people who have macular degeneration. This same tiny gene deformity may also be responsible for problems with the immune system and with a low level of chronic inflammation found in several common conditions. This knowledge is leading to new concepts of how AMD develops, but it is too soon for anyone to be tested for this gene defect since nothing can really be done if it is found and there may well be other factors at play besides heredity.

The function of genes is even more complex since each gene instructs the cell to manufacture a specific protein. This protein is determined by the cell's location. If in the liver, the protein helps make bile. If in the retina, the protein helps make rhodopsin, the vision chemical.

The process of actually putting the gene to work is accomplished by a so-called messenger strand of the gene - a single, not a double strand - called RNA (ribonucleic acid). This messenger RNA migrates from the nucleus into the cytoplasm of the cell. (It may be useful here to visualize each cell as an egg where the shell is the cell membrane, the egg white the cytoplasm, and the yolk as the nucleus.) In the cytoplasm, the messenger RNA sets up the factory to manufacturer the specific protein that the cell needs to perform its function.

If this particular cell we are examining is in a rod or cone of the retina, the protein produced may have some function in the cycle wherein opsin joins with vitamin A to form rhodopsin. If the cell is in the RPE (Retinal Pigment Epithelium), the messenger RNA may be involved with the recycling of the visual pigment or perhaps, with digesting the microscopic disks of rod and cone material that are constantly being shed in the process of seeing. One can imagine that if this "digestion" process of getting rid of parts of rods and cone cells is interfered with, the drusen can build up. These, in turn, form the basis for the inflammatory or degenerative changes in the macula. It appears more and more likely that a defect in the structure or function of the DNA or RNA in the rods, cones, or RPE cells is closely related to the cause of AMD in many cases.

Many, many genes are involved in maintaining the health of the eye and indeed every organ in the body, on a microscopic cellular level. Let me try to explain the fascinating story of the recent discovery that a tiny change (mutation) in one gene may be responsible for up to 50% of cases of AMD.

The 23 pairs of chromosomes are designated by their shape and numbered 1 through 23. On a particular spot or "locus" on chromosome number one is the gene which creates (codes for) a particular protein called Complement Factor H. Also called CFH, this protein plays a large role in the immune system's ability to reduce chronic low-level inflammation in tissues, including the retinal pigment epithelium (RPE) we discussed. It has been found that a "mistake" (mutation) can occur in one of the hundreds of amino acids which make up CFH—one common molecule, tyrosine, is replaced by another, histidine. People with this tiny alteration are seven times more likely to develop AMD than those with the usual arrangements of amino acids. I hasten to add that it is now not recommended that anyone run out and get tested for this gene, for two reasons. Number one it is very expensive and nothing can be done if it is positive. Number two, it is suggestive but not at all certain that AMD will occur in a carrier of this gene. A positive finding can therefore cause a great deal of anxiety and fear unnecessarily.

The main lesson to be learned from this fascinating genetic discovery is that this mutation, like many others, which occurs throughout our lives, can be caused or at least accelerated by smoking, ultraviolet light, chemical pollutants and obesity. Obviously, all of the above should be avoided to the maximum possible degree, as I discussed earlier.

There is another very interesting and useful piece of information connected to the gene for Complement Factor H. This molecule, CFH, is intimately associated with the C-Reactive Protein (CRP). This is the protein molecule, which is involved with low levels of chronic inflammation anywhere in the body. It is increasingly used as a blood test to determine the early presence of conditions ranging from cardiovascular disease, arthritis to macular degeneration. The CRP blood level is not specific for the disease but can alert the doctor to perform further investigations to establish a diagnosis.

New information about the genetic—not necessarily only hereditary—mechanism involved in AMD is rapidly accumulating. It is a very exciting field; stay tuned!

CHAPTER 6

Therapies

"Can AMD be cured?" This perfectly reasonable question is asked by virtually every AMD patient. After all, we live in a scientific and technical age when it seems that everything is possible.

Unfortunately, the short answer is that macular degeneration cannot be cured, at least not in the sense that we can cure vision loss from a cataract with surgery, or cure an ear infection with antibiotics.

Remember that macular degeneration involves the destruction of light-sensing nerve cells in the central retina. The body can replace lost blood or damaged skin cells, but it cannot replace dead nerve cells. That is why the effects of macular degeneration cannot be reversed. Our scotomas are a result of nerve cell loss, and once lost, those cells are gone forever. We must live with our scotomas for the rest of our lives.

So why devote an entire chapter to therapies?

Well, the fact is that the word *therapy* encompasses much more than cure. I learned this lesson from a wise professor in medical school who took the time to tell a cocky graduate that a cure is just one of four possible things that a physician can offer a patient—and is usually the least reliable of the four. It has always been that way, he said, and always will be—the same four Cs.

Nevertheless, cure is the C word that all patients want to hear first. However, contrary to common belief, this commodity is in limited supply in any field of medicine. For some conditions, such as certain tumors, gallbladder attacks, and cataracts, we have surgical cures, in which the problematic tissue or organ is removed and the patient is cured of the disability. Antibiotics are probably the best example of a medical cure, a cure in which the causative agent is eliminated. (Unfortunately, this is somewhat less so now, as many strains of bacteria are becoming resistant to antibiotics.) In a wider sense, we have cured the world of certain viral infections, such as smallpox, through the widespread use of vaccines. But when you consider the vast number of diseases that afflict mankind, from the common cold to AIDS, it is humbling to realize that for most of them—including, alas, macular degeneration—we have no cure.

That doesn't mean cures for age-related macular degeneration are not being investigated; they are, and aggressively. For instance, with heredity becoming more and more suspect as the cause of macular degeneration, the most promising route to a prevention of this disorder is that of gene therapy. This will be oriented toward preventing AMD-related vision loss in patients at high risk of developing it, not toward reversing its effects in people who already have it. Also under investigation as a therapy for a small subset of AMD patients is a delicate operation in which the retina is shifted ever so slightly so that undamaged light-sensing cells of the macula can rest on a healthy bed of nourishing retinal tissue. There are even groups working on a high-tech artificial eye that would be connected to the occipital lobe in the brain. However, as clever as all these ideas are, they are all still far outside the realm of reality and implementation. The sad fact is that an effective and reliable cure for age-related macular degeneration is not yet on the horizon; to suggest otherwise would be to extend false hope.

Compassion and Comfort

But two of the other C words, compassion and comfort, are valuable aspects of therapy that every AMD patient should expect from every physician. The doctor's demonstration of compassion—a true understanding of and empathy for the distress, pain, and anxiety that the AMD patient is experiencing—is of utmost importance in establishing a doctor-patient bond that facilitates and augments any therapy.

Comfort is also something that doctors can offer the patient with age-related macular degeneration. Most people associate comfort with alleviation of pain, but of course, with macular degeneration there is no pain. However, there *is* the aching frustration of never being able to see quite what you want to look at. A doctor who repeatedly reassures his or her patient that the world will not be erased from sight or who helps the patient to attain greater independence by means of devices, techniques, and supportive groups or agencies gives comfort. In short, the caring doctor should know all the modalities of modern low-vision rehabilitation and should provide a referral to the small but growing number of specialists in the field of low-vision rehabilitation.

One good way of finding a low-vision specialist with such characteristics is to seek a referral from agencies that specialize in assisting people with low vision. Three of the best-known such agencies are Lighthouse International, Helen Keller International, and the National Association for the Visual Handicapped. (Contact information may be found in Resources.)

Control

The fourth C word, and the one most applicable to

age-related macular degeneration, is control. This is the focus of most of the current research into therapy for macular degeneration. Indeed, control is the major function in most areas of medicine, since the most common modern Western diseases—hypertension, cardiovascular disease, diabetes, arthritis, asthma, allergies, gastrointestinal diseases, and glaucoma—can only be controlled, not cured, by modern medicine. (It is true that the control, by halting the progress of the disease and preventing symptoms or disability, has an effect similar to a cure in some instances. In most cases, however, the patient and doctor are both painfully aware that constant regimen of medication and management is essential to prevent serious outbreaks.)

Only Wet AMD Can Be Treated, and Only in Some Cases

Virtually all efforts to control age-related macular degeneration are at best effective only for the wet form of AMD, in which fluid leaking from abnormal blood vessels under the macula leads to the destruction of the macula's light-sensing nerve cells. You may recall from chapter 4 that the wet form of the disease accounts for only about 10 percent of all AMD cases. For such patients, new surgical and medical treatments show great promise for slowing or stopping the progression of the disease. For AMD patients with the so-called dry form of the disease, the most promising ways to control AMD may be through nutrition, discussed in chapter 7.

At the Horizon

Since the first edition of this book was published in 2000, there has been a dramatic rise in the treatment options available for wet, or neovascular, AMD. In my original chapter on treatment, I discussed a number of possibilities, which I will recount now both for historical interest and to demonstrate how the rapid pace of medical research transforms our thinking.

The original gold standard of treatment, argon laser photocoagulation, is no longer used at all due to the possibility of collateral retinal damage. A new therapy under research at the time utilizing a very mild laser treatment of any drusen present has been shown to be ineffective. External beam radiation focused carefully on bleeding areas has completely fallen into disuse. Various highly intricate surgical procedures involving the retina are now considered only in very few cases because of relatively high complication rates.

The technique of photodynamic therapy, or PDT, was heralded with great hope and fanfare and indeed was quite successful in sealing off leaking or newly forming tiny blood vessels. This technique, using an intravenous drug, verteporforin, caused clotting and occlusion within the abnormal vessels when they were exposed to a very weak laser light. This technique is still selectively used, not alone (mono therapy) but in conjunction with the new "gold standard," anti-VEGF injections into the eye.

To help you understand this new treatment, I must first explain the acronym VEGF (pronounced vedg-ef). It stands for Vascular Endothelial Growth Factor and is involved in a very important function in our bodies called angiogenesis. This process of forming new blood vessels takes place normally in healing injuries, and abnormally in causing cancers to grow. The tiny new blood vessels begin to grow in response to a chemical enzyme the body cells produce: VEGF.

When the new blood vessel growth acts in a way which can cause further damage to our bodies, such as helping cancers grow and spread or forming new, tiny vessels under the retina where they can bleed, we would like to inhibit and stop that growth. This is where anti-VEGF drugs come into play. These newly developed drugs, commercially named Macugen, Lucentis and Avastin, can block the effects of VEGF in the cells of the artery wall and thereby prevent the beginning formation of new blood vessels.

Unfortunately, in diseases of the retina like AMD, the drug must be placed near the retina and cannot be given as a pill or an intravenous injection. A small amount of it must be injected directly into the eyeball at frequent intervals, usually once a month.

Although the image of an injection into the eye disturbs many people, the procedure of intravitreal injection, when done properly with a tiny needle, can be almost painless with extremely few complications.

It has been shown that when treatment is started early, before severe leakage from new tiny blood vessels, vision can be preserved and in some cases even slightly improved.

In summary, present day treatment consists of the anti-VEGF drugs, usually Avastin or Lucentis being injected directly into the vitreous gel within the eyeball at regular intervals until all bleeding or leakage has stopped. Until the next breakthrough, everyone with wet AMD should feel comfortable with this treatment if it is recommended by the ophthalmologist.

As for the majority of patients with dry AMD, there is increasing interest in the nutritional control of progression and a few other investigational therapies. The three more interesting ones I have studied are the following: First, a new drug, commercially named Copaxone, currently used in cases of multiple sclerosis, is being tested to determine if it may slow the progression of dry AMD in addition to preventing the conversion of the dry form to the more disabling wet form of AMD. Second, an experimental drug labeled POT-4 is being tested for its ability to reduce "complement activation," the process which sets up local inflammation and VEGF activity in retinal cells. Third, another drug under investigation and labeled OT-551 may protect the retinal pigment cells (RPE) from oxidative damage and block angiogenesis stimulated by VEGF.

Therapeutic possibilities are many and exciting. Let's hope they are realized soon.

Hope for the Future

What all of the therapies covered in this chapter have in common is that they are under investigation within the confines of the scientific method. Studies are being carefully constructed, and the results will be published and subjected to peer review by other researchers. This is really the only way to ensure that new drugs and surgical procedures are both effective and safe.

Regrettably, other drugs and procedures now being promoted as AMD therapies have *not* been tested by the scientific method. These procedures, some of which include so-called blood cleansing, are often aggressively advertised by their practitioners as cures for age-related macular degeneration. Although they are understandably attractive to the AMD patient desperate for improved vision, I am highly skeptical about the value of any "miracle cure" that has not been analyzed in a controlled and peer-reviewed clinical study. If you are considering a costly procedure based on an advertisement, a celebrity endorsement, or the experience of a friend of a friend of a friend, please ask for and heed the advice of your ophthalmologist first.

Meanwhile, if this chapter seems inconclusive and a bit confusing, it is because that is the current status of therapy for age-related macular degeneration. But so much work is being done by so many talented, dedicated people that more effective therapies will undoubtedly be found someday.

In addition, one aspect of self-help has been decidedly underemphasized by many ophthalmologists and retinal specialists: the role that nutrition may play in preventing or forestalling the onset of age-related macular degeneration, and possibly in slowing its progress among those who already have it. Chapter 7 details the current knowledge of nutritional and dietary therapy, and offers my personal recommendations in this area.

CHAPTER 7

The Role of Nutrition

"First, do no harm." That's from the Hippocratic oath, taken by every doctor for generations. And it is why I can confidently recommend that everyone with age-related macular degeneration eat a diet rich in spinach and vitamins C and E. Such a dietary regimen may very well help preserve your eyesight, but even if it doesn't, it certainly will do you no harm.

In fact, though, the evidence that dietary changes can be helpful for people with age-related macular degeneration has become very compelling. Of course, no amount of spinach, vitamins, or other nutritional supplements will improve your vision by shrinking your central blind spot. Your scotoma is caused by the loss of light-sensing nerve cells, and these cells cannot be repaired or replaced no matter what you eat. However, what proper nutrition may be able to do is to slow down or prevent the *worsening* of your vision.

In order to understand the role of nutrition in age-related macular degeneration, you must first understand the process of oxidation, the roles that free radicals and antioxidants play in retinal health, and the importance to your vision of certain chemicals that are found in abundance in spinach and other leafy green vegetables.

Antioxidants and Macular Degeneration

In the normal function of any cell in the body, the specific work, or oxidation, of the cell generates waste products, molecules that have an odd number of electrons rather than a stable even number. These molecules are called free radicals; they can link with other molecules such as proteins, fats, oxygen, or even DNA in the nucleus of the cell. This joining together damages the existing normal molecule.

The production of free radicals increases naturally as part of the aging process. In the retina, free radicals are also produced by the impact of light rays, particularly in the ultraviolet to blue part of the spectrum. Fortunately, the body has a protective mechanism that helps control the free radicals. The so-called protective or scavenger molecules in the cell join with, or gobble up, the noxious free radicals before they can interact with the more vital proteins and lipids. Some of these scavenger molecules are vitamin E, vitamin C, selenium and, in the eye particularly, lutein and zeaxanthin. In other words, the normal amount of vitamin C, E, and lutein in the lens of the eye usually helps protect the clear lens fibers from becoming cloudy and forming a cataract.

The lutein in the macula and the surrounding retinal pigment epithelium may also protect the rods and cones and cells of the retinal pigment epithelium. They probably do this in two ways. First, they prevent the free radicals from interacting with the rich lipid layer in the retinal pigment epithelium, thereby reducing the amount of fatty substance that may cause more drusen. Second, the yellowish color of the lutein may actually absorb more of the bluish light that strikes the retina and may cause more photooxidative (light-induced) damage to the delicate macula cells.

Oxidation

Consider what happens when you cut an apple in half and allow it to stand exposed to the air, where it comes in contact with oxygen. The flesh of the apple turns brown. This is a result of a process called oxidation. Oxidation is the chemical process by which cells use oxygen to create energy. When oxygen is added to a molecule of fat, protein, or carbohydrate, a chemical reaction ensues that liberates energy for the cell to continue its work. In the case of the apple, the brown discoloration of the flesh results from the oxidation of the fruit's sugar molecules. Now consider the effect of spreading lemon juice on the flesh of the apple immediately after it is cut open. It doesn't turn brown. The reason is that the ascorbic acid in the lemon prevents oxidation. Another way of saying this is that the ascorbic acid, also known as vitamin C, acts as an antioxidant.

One natural result of the oxidation process is the production of free radicals, which are molecules made unstable by a change in their atomic structure. These free radicals are missing an electron; in an attempt to correct their unbalanced atomic state, they attempt to steal electrons from the atoms of other cells. Left unchecked, the chemical reactions caused by free radicals can lead to a variety of harmful effects in the body, including damage to the delicate cells of the retina.

After they are produced, most free radicals are destroyed quickly by the body's natural antioxidants, which are molecules that gobble up the free radicals. But if the body does not have enough of these natural antioxidants to control the free radicals, we need additional antioxidants from nutritional supplements, mainly vitamins C and E.

The Importance of Plant Chemicals

Lutein and zeaxanthin are two chemicals in the family of carotenoids, compounds found in plants whose function is to protect plant cells from light damage. In the macula, these chemicals appear to prevent the oxidation of lipids (fat) in the cell membrane. These oxidized lipids could lead to the accumulation of the waste product called drusen, which is always associated with age-related macular degeneration.

In addition, lutein, which provides the yellowish color to the macula, appears to inhibit damage from the blue light of the electromagnetic spectrum. It does this by absorbing blue light, which may be damaging to the macula.

Spinach, kale, and other green leafy vegetables are excellent sources of lutein, but it is also available as a dietary supplement. While lutein is available now in pharmacies and health-food stores, it is probably somewhat preferable to consume it as a food source, since some other agents may not be included in the supplements.

Establishing the Connection Between Nutrition and AMD

A quiet revolution in scientific thinking about the role of nutrition in macular disease has been going on since 1945, when Nobel Prize laureate George Wald first recognized the presence of lutein in the macula of the eye. More recently, numerous articles in the *Archives of Ophthalmology* have identified risk factors for age-related macular degeneration that include insufficient levels of vitamin C, vitamin E, selenium, and zinc, as well as high cholesterol and smoking. In addition, other studies have shown that a high level of blood lutein is associated with a significant decrease in the risk of developing age-related macular degeneration.

The defining event in the AMD "nutrition revolution" came with the publication of the November 9, 1994 *Journal of the American Medical Association*. Dr. Johanna Seddon and her associates at the Massachusetts Eye and Ear Infirmary and Harvard University studied a large number of people with age-related macular degeneration alongside a group of people from the same age group without AMD. They compared the two groups' dietary intake of carotenoids (mainly lutein and zeaxanthin) in dark green leafy vegetables, as well as their consumption of vitamins C and E. The article's brief introduction and its conclusion should serve as a wake-up call to patients and eye care professionals alike:

> There is increasing speculation that dietary factors, particularly antioxidants, may prevent or impede the progression of AMD. The theory is biologically plausible. The outer retina, rich in polyunsaturated fatty acids, may be altered adversely by "free radical" production and oxidation and, conversely, may be protected by nutrients

that block this oxidative damage. Anti-oxidants may also help to maintain the integrity of the ... blood vessels that supply the macular region of the retina.

[The article's conclusion:] Increasing the consumption of foods rich in certain carotenoids, in particular dark green leafy vegetables, may decrease the risk of developing advanced or exudative AMD, the most visually disabling form of macular degeneration among older people.

My own feeling about age-related macular degeneration is that it is related to a weak or abnormal gene that becomes damaged or activated over many years by a variety of toxic, environmental, dietary, metabolic, or other factors. I believe that the ensuing genetic dysfunction is aided and abetted by the action of free radicals in the retinal cells. The genetic dysfunction and the effects of the free radicals interfere with the normal "digestive" process of the retina in eliminating macular waste products. And it is the build-up of waste products that leads to the creation of drusen, which may be related to the onset of age-related macular degeneration.

The AREDS Report

In 2001, a very influential report was issued in the Archives of Ophthalmology. It was called the "Age Related Eye Disease Study," and it is known to every ophthalmologist as the AREDS Report. It detailed, in the best scientific manner, a large, national, and controlled double-blind study that a particular dose of vitamin C, vitamin E, beta carotene and zinc with copper resulted in a dramatic reduction of progression from moderate wet AMD to an advanced form of the disease.

Since that time, many ophthalmologists are recommending that all their patients with AMD take some version of this mix of vitamins and antioxidants. They are sold as PreserVision, Ocuvite, I-Caps and other brands.

In addition, there is a new nationwide study going on called AREDS-II. This study is adding lutein and omega-3 fish oil capsules to the basic formula. These two chemicals should give further support to the macular cells, but results will not be analyzed and published until 2011 or later. So here is a secret tip: I am advising many of my patients to add 6mg of lutein and 1000mg of fish oil to their daily AREDS routine. There are few if any downside risks, and if it turns out to be beneficial, you've gained a few years of health.

So What Should You Do?

I recommend the following approach:

• Take a comprehensive multivitamin/multimineral preparation. This should be taken one time each day, regularly and permanently. The basic formulation of brand name products is identical to most reputable generics. These preparations contain 100 percent of the daily value (DV) of most major vitamins, as well as adequate amounts of the trace minerals also essential to a healthy metabolic state. It is amazing to me to find that a significant number, perhaps a majority, of older people do not take a daily multivitamin! There is considerable evidence that the diet of many seniors, especially those living alone, is grossly deficient in variety and nutritional value. In addition, there are organic changes with age that interfere with the absorption of certain important vitamins, particularly vitamin B_{12}.

• Take supplemental vitamin B_{12}. I test all my older patients with a simple balance test: Stand on one foot for longer than five seconds. This is probably an over-simplified test for our kinesthetic sense, a sense mediated by end organs located in muscles, tendons, and joints and stimulated by bodily movements and tensions. A large number of people over age sixty-five fail this test, which may be related, at least in part, to a decreased blood level of vitamin B_{12}. This vitamin is essential to the normal formation of red blood cells and to building up the myelin sheath, or covering, of nerve fibers. A surprising 30 percent of patients who are over the age of sixty-five may have a vitamin B_{12} deficiency. This is due to a change in the stomach lining with age that stops production of a chemical needed to absorb B_{12} from food. I recommend 100 micrograms daily to help maintain a normally functioning neurological and blood-forming system.

• The big hitter in macular therapy is the carotenoid chemicals, mostly lutein and zeaxanthine. Carotenoids are a major class of compounds found in fresh fruits and vegetables, and they are powerful antioxidants. The important carotenoids include beta-carotene, found in large amounts in carrots, kale, and spinach; lutein and zeaxanthine in kale, spinach, and broccoli; and lycopene, found mostly in tomatoes.

Lutein is particularly important because it is absorbed from these foods and transported in relatively large quantities to the macula and the lens of the eye. In each of these areas it has a specific, helpful antioxidant action. It appears that ingested lutein may indeed lower the risk of developing age-related macular degeneration and even cataracts. There are also new studies indicating that ingested lutein might prevent the advancement of AMD in people who are mildly to moderately impaired.

To consume enough lutein, you should eat as much spinach and kale as you can enjoy and take either lutein tablets of at least 6 milligrams three times a day, usually derived from purified extracts of marigold flowers, or lutein in the form of concentrated spinach, also three tablets a day. Lutein supplements, such as Ocuguard Plus (which also includes other antioxidants), can be found in many drugstores and vitamin stores and can be ordered from health food catalogues or the Internet. Two sources are listed in the Appendix.

Other Nutritional Supplements

For those who wish to go even further with nutrition, there are certain herbal or mineral compounds that may—repeat, *may*—be helpful. First, though, a warning. Interest is soaring in alternative therapies for many diseases. Some of these therapies involve herbs and other compounds that, in smaller moderate amounts, may indeed be helpful. Others may have no effect, and some—particularly if taken in large quantities—can have harmful effects. As a physician with a strong background in the scientific method, I am hesitant to recommend any therapy that has not been proven safe and effective in large, well-conducted clinical studies. However, there are instances where conducting such studies are not practical. For instance, altering the diet of a large group of people to assess the effects of the change on their health is not ethical. In cases where there is strong evidence that a dietary supplement is helpful and not particularly risky, I recommend that my patients use it if they wish. Those that I feel fall into this category are:

• Selenium, an essential trace mineral that appears to increase production of an important bodily antioxidant, glutathione peroxidase, which is particularly important in the prevention of cataracts. The usual suggested supplement is 100 to 200 micrograms. (This amount should not be exceeded because at high doses there might be some toxic effects.)

• Zinc, which is also an essential trace element in the human metabolism. The absorption of zinc appears to decrease as we age. It appears to play an important role in maintaining the body's immune reaction to germs and illness. It also acts as an important antioxidant. While it is believed to be particularly useful in macular function, that ability has not been corroborated. It may still be useful, but you should not exceed 15 to 30 milligrams because higher doses, particularly those over 100 milligrams, can be damaging in other ways. Excess zinc can deplete copper storage in the body, leading to a copper deficiency anemia.

The alternative medicine/health-food industry has many other suggested "remedies" for eye disease. These include bilberry extracts, garlic, quercetin, coenzyme Q10, glutathione, omega-3 fish oils, and several other ground-up raw herbs. Unfortunately, none of these has been subjected to the clinical trials needed to determine efficacy. Many of them are harmless, but a recent report in the *New England Journal of Medicine* indicates that a few alternative medicines, perhaps overused or even adulterated, have resulted in serious injury or even death. A maxim I learned in medical school still applies: "Be not the first to try the new, nor the last to discard the old."

In summary, I advise you to adopt a well-rounded diet rich in fresh fruits and vegetables, plus take the following daily:

- Full-strength multivitamin/multimineral tablet

- Vitamin E, 400 IU

- Vitamin C, 500 milligrams, sustained-release form

- Vitamin B_{12}, 100 micrograms

- Purified lutein, at least 6 milligrams three times a day, or the equivalent in concentrated spinach pills

If you want to know my personal daily vitamin and supplement routine, it is:

- Multivitamin/mineral, one per day

- Preservision capsule, two per day

- Lutein capsule, one per day

- Fish oil omega-3 capsule, 1,000 milligrams, one per day

- Vitamin B_{12}, 100 micrograms, one per day

- Vitamin D3, 400 IU, two per day

Important for You *and* Your Children

One final note on the importance of nutrition. As I said at the outset of this chapter, no amount of antioxidants and lutein will reverse the damage to your vision. The hope is that by adopting these recommendations you may slow the progression of your AMD. But there is yet another reason for paying attention to this information on nutrition, and it concerns your children. If, as we suspect, the propensity to develop macular degeneration is inherited, then your children are at risk of developing it as they age. By urging them to adopt a vegetable-rich diet heavy in antioxidant vitamins and lutein, you may be helping them reduce their risk of developing age-related macular degeneration. And in any event, you certainly will be doing them no harm.

CHAPTER 8

It's About More Than Vision

The central blind spot that is the hallmark of age-related macular degeneration threatens to cloud much more than your eyesight. Particularly when we first learn about the irrevocability of our disease, many of us feel that the scotoma casts a shadow over our entire sense of self. It's easy to feel overwhelmed by a cascade of fears about all sorts of losses: reading, work, travel, leisure, friendships, and most of all, independence. I've given these losses a great deal of thought and have found that it helps to list them along with relevant remedies.

Loss of Ease and Pleasure in Reading

For the person with age-related macular degeneration, reading is usually never as easy and enjoyable as it used to be. Indeed, the ability to read material without effort is often the first loss recognized by the patient with AMD, and may be first noticed when you find it hard to decipher the mail, the newspaper, or the prices on a supermarket shelf.

Addressing the Loss

If you want to continue reading, you can. Virtually everyone with age-related macular degeneration can continue to enjoy books, newspapers, and magazines for as long as they want to. Many people find that they can read quite well simply by learning to hold their reading material closer to their eyes. Others use large-print or audiotape versions of books and periodicals, which are readily available at most good public libraries.

At some point, you may find great benefit from one or more of the many low-vision aids that are widely available. (See Resources for listings of companies that provide such aids.) A skilled low-vision therapist can help you select the proper device and provide valuable instruction in its precise use. You may need help to determine, for example, whether a hand or spectacle-mounted magnifier is preferable, or if, as in many cases, both are needed. In addition, the quality of the optics of the lens is an important factor, and cheaper is not necessarily just as good.

For those whose reading ability is still compromised with even well chosen devices, a technique called eccentric viewing can greatly improve the ease of reading. This is a process of essentially seeing around the scotoma. If you look just slightly to one side or the other of what you really want to see, the image of that which you want to see becomes more visible because it is seen by means of the rods and cones at the edge of the macula. It takes time and practice to learn to do this, but it has been shown to significantly benefit many people with low-vision reading problems.

A small minority of AMD patients may find it useful to invest in higher-end technology to help them with their reading. These devices include elaborate closed-circuit television systems, which project a highly magnified image of the reading matter onto a television screen or computer monitor. Also helpful are the latest voice synthesizer reading machines, which have come down in price enough so that they are within the reach of many people. The ability of these devices to "read" any material fed into them will make their relatively high cost seem a good investment for the relatively few AMD patients who may need them.

Loss of Ease of Spoken Communication

Sadly, age-related macular degeneration frequently occurs in the same age group that is undergoing presbyacusis, a moderate age-related hearing loss. In addition, we are all much more dependent than we realize on observing people's mouths and facial expressions or body language when they talk. These visible clues to the subtleties of meaning—humor, sarcasm, etc.—are largely unavailable to a person with a moderate central blind spot in each eye. In addition, the inability to promptly recognize faces and objects can lead to a mistaken impression of unfriendliness on the part of others.

Addressing the Loss

If the effect of AMD is exacerbated by a hearing defect, the hearing loss should be corrected, if possible, by an appropriate hearing aid. Having said this, I must add that many people who do indeed have a hearing loss resist doing anything about it.

If hearing loss is not an issue, you might find it useful to practice an eccentric viewing skill that can be very helpful in overcoming the loss of ease in spoken communication. This technique is more easily mastered than the eccentric viewing skill needed for reading. Try the following exercise. Look directly at the head of a person as if it were the face of a clock. Next, transfer the center of your gaze at or above the twelve o'clock point while maintaining the whole of your mental attention on analyzing facial expression. After a few seconds, move on to stare at the one o'clock position, then the two o'clock position, and so on. Try to compare the points and determine which position gave you the best general view of the face.

That position is your preferred viewing fixation point. When that point is established, always look at people and objects by focusing on that position, while at the same time concentrating sharply on the details of the target object. This approach can be very rewarding if it is practiced and becomes automatic.

Loss of the Techniques of Daily Living

One's self-image, along with the actual image one presents to society, can be adversely affected by minor difficulties. Macular degeneration makes it difficult to apply makeup, to shave properly, to recognize when items of clothing are soiled, and to know when fingernails need cleaning. A routine task such as cooking can become frustrating because it is difficult to see the proper oven temperature or the lines on a measuring cup. These difficulties can aggravate your sense of loss of independence. Furthermore, because you are likely to encounter new difficulties periodically rather than all at once, you may, like many people, mistakenly assume that each new difficulty signifies a deterioration of your vision.

Addressing the Loss

For most household tasks, specific optical and non-optical aids can help. Magnifying mirrors, very bright lights, and established cleaning routines may all be necessary. Gadgets are available that enable you to feel elevated marks on a measuring scale or on an oven knob. These and many others can be obtained through a number of sources, some of which are identified in the Appendix. In a broader sense, when a new difficulty arises, it should be regarded as a challenge to overcome rather than a cause to panic. Usually, a difficulty not previously identified is due to its not having been encountered. It does not necessarily mean that your macular degeneration has progressed. Attempting to assess the progression of your AMD based on your success, or lack thereof, in performing the tasks of daily living is fruitless and depressing. Rely on your eye doctor for such assessment.

Loss of Mobility

It is not just the ability to drive safely that deteriorates along with the macula. Many AMD patients find that their scotoma, or central blind spot, also interferes with their walking or using public transportation, thereby limiting their ability to get around and isolating them. For someone with advanced macular degeneration, for instance, it would be quite difficult to identify a bus by number or decipher the small print of a train schedule. Walking may pose problems with: curbs, cracks, and red lights or signs.

Addressing the Loss

Far and away the most wrenching problem for everyone with age-related macular degeneration is the need to curtail or eliminate driving. (The question of when to stop driving is the subject of chapter 9.) Unquestionably, the inability to drive poses huge problems in independent daily living. Having to rely on relatives, friends, senior transportation services, or public transportation is inconvenient, restricting, and for some, humiliating. You must find the inner strength required to avoid becoming shut in by your condition. This takes determination, but you may well find that the rewards of leading as active a life as possible are more-than-fair compensation for dealing with the challenges posed by the inability to drive.

The other issue in mobility concerns independent travel, which can definitely be helped by the use of pocket telescopes and magnifiers. I think everyone with visual impairment should carry one of each. The magnifier can be used to read schedules, maps, and other printed matter. The pocket telescope, generally one to three inches in length, is extremely useful to spot street signs, bus or train routes, and directions at street crossings. Although you may find using these devises awkward, time-consuming, and even embarrassing, they facilitate progress from isolation and self-pity to a greater level of mobility and independence.

Loss of Confidence in the Remaining Senses

Throughout life, we use our vision to validate our other senses. When we hear a sound, we immediately look toward it to determine its origin. If food smells or tastes bad, we inspect it for signs of spoilage. The mildest itch or cut or casual touch is carefully examined. When age-related vision loss is accompanied by age-related loss of hearing, smell, and taste, a loss of confidence in one's senses can lead to a loss of confidence in one's self.

Addressing the Loss

Hearing, the sensory loss that most often accompanies the visual loss of age-related macular degeneration, usually can be compensated for technologically. I routinely do a screening audiometry test on my patients, and I urge those who show the high frequency hearing loss of presbyacusis to seek audiological assistance. The age-related loss of acuteness in the sense of smell and taste are much less often involved and do not often become a problem. Deterioration in the sensory pathway that helps maintain balance, however, can pose additional problems for individuals with age-related macular degeneration. This kinesthetic sense—the messages to the brain from the muscles, tendons, and joints about where we are in space— may be impaired by the faulty absorption of vitamin B_{12}, which often occurs in the elderly. For this reason, as I mentioned earlier, I frequently prescribe an extra daily dose of vitamin B_{12}, usually 100 micrograms, to help prevent any unsteadiness of gait, which would certainly be aggravated by a visual loss.

Loss of Pleasurable Vision

Those who derive pleasure and excitement from art in museums, from viewing photographs of loved ones, or from appreciating nature or beautiful crafts may be very distressed by loss of the ability to appreciate texture, design, detail, nuance, and color.

Addressing the Loss

Each of us must come to grips with how far we are willing to go to maintain pleasures that are not necessities. For instance, to experience the brilliance of a painting's color and texture you could use a combination of a binocular telescope for overall viewing and a magnifier for closer inspection. This will give you at least a partial sense of the beauty to be observed. While it may not be what it was to us before our decreased visual acuity, with effort it still can be a thrill. Visually detailed hobbies can be aided by telemicroscopes and loupes. You will have to determine for yourself in each case whether it is worth the effort to overcome the difficulty with technical means. Of course it can be done, but you must overcome denial, inertia, embarrassment, and depression to achieve the pleasurable experiences in life to which we all aspire.

Loss of Recreation

As distinguished from visual pleasures, recreation implies participating in what is viewed. Although your ability to engage in sports, games, and hobbies may not be completely lost, the increased difficulty in dealing with details can limit your enjoyment of these activities. Plays, movies, television, sporting events—all may be difficult to fully experience. This can make us feel less relaxed and more depressed.

Addressing the Loss

Visual aids can help greatly with these activities, but again, individual motivation will determine which activities are pursued, and how actively. I remember a patient of mine who had a severe visual loss. Charles had retinitis pigmentosa, a hereditary disease that by age sixty had forced him to use a cane to feel his way. With a visual field of about 5 degrees, rather than the normal 160 degrees or more, he was essentially blind. Yet he helped create a sport called BeeperBall, baseball for the really visually handicapped, and he played it extensively. The ball emits a loud tone and is followed and hit by auditory clues. It is now a national sport that is enjoyed by many.

I mention Charles to indicate the broad spectrum of activities available to those with a much less severe visual handicap. Everyone should maintain or start pleasurable activities, with visual aids if needed, to have a positive outlook on life. This has been shown to yield not only psychological benefits but also overall physiological improvement as well. What hobbies, interests, passions do you love? Don't give them up— find ways to enjoy them.

Loss of Financial Security

For those of us who were still employed when AMD struck, we must face the likelihood of an earlier-than-expected retirement, along with a subsequent reduction of income. In addition, provisions must be made for increased medical bills, higher transportation costs, and additional household help. Many find it difficult to read bills, write checks, and follow the details of one's assets. All of this can induce a heightened sense of financial hardship.

Addressing the Loss

The average patient with AMD is in or near retirement. If you've planned for retirement, a major source of anxiety is at least removed. Where family support is available, additional comfort is provided. This does not mean that the sense of financial insecurity is eliminated. On the contrary, even with an adequate income, the fear of ever-increasing needs with diminishing vision induces a sense of financial vulnerability. Here are four sources of comfort in this area:

• There is no reason that a physically capable person with age-related macular degeneration cannot pursue gainful employment if he or she wants or needs to. Certainly, the issue of sparing the eyes by not using them should be disposed of again. If a person with macular degeneration can function in his or her job or be trained for another, there is absolutely no medical reason why he or she should not continue to work. Another way to bolster retirement income is to take on more limited tasks such as child care, babysitting, and tutoring, jobs that can be rewarding personally as well as financially.

• Each state has a commission for the blind or some other social service agency specifically concerned with those who are visually impaired. These agencies are limited to working with certain populations, such as the legally blind, and within certain parameters. By and large, they provide financial and social support services to those who qualify for assistance. Contact information can usually be found in the state government listings of the phone book.

• A number of private, voluntary agencies and foundations, such as Lighthouse International and the National Association for the Visually Handicapped, may offer financial assistance. Listings of locally based support organizations may be found in the yellow pages under "Social Service Organizations" or on the Internet.

• Last but not least is the benefit offered by the IRS on the income tax form, provided for those who qualify within the guidelines of legal blindness.

Loss of Sense of Self

A person with a vision loss no longer has the same identity as he or she once did. Your visual disability may make you feel you are unable to function in a sighted society. This different "self" is often plagued by fear of a progressive loss into total blindness. Although baseless, this fear fosters a self-image of a poor, handicapped, pathetic figure.

Addressing the Loss

We all see ourselves functioning in our own worlds of family, jobs, friends and play in a very specific manner. This image of ourselves is usually based on our life before vision loss, an image that must unhappily be brought up-to-date. Most people can adapt to the new lifestyle and self-image. However, you must work to dispell your fear of increasing or total blindness. In addition, you should seek out self-help groups of people with age-related macular degeneration, through which you can share your fears and draw inspiration from others.

Loss of Independence and Self-Esteem

This is the crux of the issue. After all, the hallmark of maturity is the ability to do things for yourself or others *by yourself*. From the first time you have to ask someone, "Would you read that telephone number for me?" you fear an inexorably progressive loss of independence. This can lead you to an abrupt transition from leading life with a mature and capable feeling to suddenly feeling aged and frail, even if you are only slightly over sixty-five years of age. In fact, you may also start brooding about mortality, which leads to the depression so commonly seen with age-related macular degeneration. When this loss of identity is associated, as it often is, with the loss of your career, it may bring about a profound drop in your self-esteem and an increase in your feelings of uselessness and inadequacy.

Addressing the Loss

You are far more than just your sight. There is a considerable body of psychological and philosophical evidence that we validate ourselves through relationships with others. Certainly your independence may have to evolve, in a few areas, into codependence. But these new codependencies—whether they are with a spouse, friend, sibling, child, grandchild or companion—can be deeply enriching for everyone involved if they lead to new opportunities for sharing thoughts, memories, and time.

You must break the connection between independence and self-esteem. To realize that the two are unconnected, one need only think of Professor Stephen Hawking, the world-famous physicist, who is not only confined to a wheelchair but also unable to speak clearly. We can also draw inspiration from Christopher Reeve, the talented actor who became paralyzed in a tragic riding accident. Hawking displays a strength of self that transcends his near-total physical incapacity, as did Reeve prior to his death in 2004. Most of us do not have genius or star status, but we all have a capacity to be of value to others and ourselves that transcends the five senses.

Finally, you must try to recognize and complete all the stages of grieving that typically accompany the loss of vision. These stages of grief are comparable to mourning the loss of a loved one or to receiving the diagnosis of a terminal illness. The first stage is denial or disbelief: "It's not true that my vision is worse." Second, there is desperation—a flight to any clinic, city, or country that might offer even the smallest chance of help. The third stage is depression, which frequently sets in when the first two stages are played out. It is perfectly normal to feel frightened, alone, sad, depressed, or hopeless, as long as that stage ultimately progresses to the next, fourth stage: acceptance. This, in turn, is just the beginning of the drive toward physical and spiritual rehabilitation, which becomes complete with the fifth stage, transcendence. This final stage, achieved after we pass through the others, allows us to see that we can use adversity to gain a level of insight, understanding—and yes, even excitement in simply living—that we might not have been capable of without the misfortune.

It's About Perception

This chapter is entitled, "It's About More Than Vision." The subtitle should be "It's about perception." After all, a great deal of both problem and resolution comes down to just that: perception. Difficulties with visual loss are certainly real and initially devastating. But at the risk of sounding trite, I must reaffirm my view that life is vastly more complex and wonderful than what we can see, as miraculous as sight is.

A person with macular degeneration remains a responsible, intelligent, mostly independent individual, giving and receiving love, help, and guidance. Great pleasure in life's experiences, spiritual fulfillment, joy, and intellectual discovery are not dependent solely on good vision. Those with a visual handicap must work around it so they can gain the ability that everyone should strive for: *Carpe diem!* Seize the day! See beyond the clouds!

CHAPTER 9

When Should You Stop Driving?

Driving is probably the toughest issue facing everyone with age-related macular degeneration. Driving is so important to our ability to function in our community, to our independence, and to our sense of self-worth that many of us with age-related macular degeneration address the issue only with the greatest reluctance.

Indeed, in working with AMD patients I have learned to postpone the discussion about driving for as long as possible in the initial interview. First I resolve more easily remedied problems with near- and far-vision aids and get to know and understand the patient better before I grapple with what is invariably a pivotal and profoundly disturbing decision.

However, because it is dangerous to drive with impaired vision, the question of driving must be tackled directly.

The answer to the question of when to stop driving, in brief, is either when you no longer can meet your state's minimum vision standards for driving or when you and your loved ones no longer feel confident about your ability to drive safely.

Know the Requirements in Your State

Minimum vision requirements for driving vary from state to state, so it is important to know the requirements in your state. Most states have a two-part vision requirement, one for visual field (side vision) and one for visual acuity (the ability to discern objects from a distance). Most AMD patients have no problem passing the visual field requirement; it is the visual acuity requirement—typically 20/40 in the better eye with glasses—where the problem arises. (See the sidebar at the end of this chapter for a list of states and their vision requirements.)

Your measurement of visual acuity is not necessarily a very good indicator of your functional visual ability. An AMD patient with 20/400 vision may cope beautifully with many of the tasks of daily life. Meanwhile, someone with a smaller scotoma and 20/70 vision may be distraught because his or her driving ability has been limited.

Of course, it is impossible to know if one's vision has deteriorated past the minimum legal driving requirements without an eye exam. Thus, many AMD patients may consciously or unconsciously put off a checkup for fear that they will fail their vision exam and be forced to stop driving. In addition, many states do not require a vision check upon license renewal, and even in those that do, the period between renewals may be long enough that one's vision could fall below the legal limits well before renewal time.

This is why it is relatively uncommon for AMD patients to find themselves being told by their ophthalmologist or a clerk at the motor vehicles bureau that they must stop driving. Most people with age-related macular degeneration need to make the decision about when to stop driving for themselves.

The Importance of Driving

This decision is unquestionably one of the most difficult that the individual with age-related macular degeneration will have to make. The ability to drive to any place for any purpose at any time is tied so firmly to our sense of an independent "self" that being deprived of this power can reduce the strongest of us to a feeling of utter helplessness.

In modern communities there are certainly alternatives to driving—a spouse, a friend, a taxi, a bus, or a community driving service. Of course, none offer the convenience of driving. But in any case, the issue is not simply one of getting from one place to another whenever you wish. The decision to stop driving is a personal and public proclamation that you have become less independent, less "capable," and more reliant on others.

The issue is particularly traumatic because of the conflict between the need to drive and the counter-vailing desire not to put oneself and others at risk by driving with impaired vision. Indeed, this is why AMD patients often quite willingly give up night driving as soon as it becomes even slightly apparent that driving in the dark is harder than it used to be.

I can relate to these feelings. Earlier in the progression of my own condition, when I could still drive by using my then-functional right eye, I would sometimes test myself while at a stop sign or red light. When I momentarily closed my good eye, I could recognize the problems I would face if the vision in that eye deteriorated further.

I remember quickly putting those thoughts about a non-driving future aside. I felt that I could probably continue driving for some time even if the vision in my good right eye declined to the level of my bad left eye. After all, I thought, I'd still be able to see the gross—albeit, distorted—image of cars, and the center line would still be visible to me, even if it might appear a bit crooked. I figured this would enable me to safely make a few local trips a week, to the post office, the supermarket, and the bank—enough driving to manage my personal affairs by myself.

I'll return to my own story in a moment, but first let me explain why I was wrong.

Vision and Driving

It is the size, density, and location of the blind spot that determines our driving capability. Safe driving requires alertness and awareness tied to rapid reflexes. After all, the unexpected event, not the expected, leads to an accident. If an unexpected event occurs in the road within the area obscured or distorted by a driver's blind spot, the driver might not react appropriately in time to avoid an accident. Surprises are possible even on a familiar road or a quiet suburban street. If our view of a pedestrian stepping into the roadway from between two parked cars, or a child on a bicycle pedaling out of a driveway, is obscured or distorted for even an instant, tragedy is inevitable.

Telescopic Driving Aids

At this point some reader is surely thinking, "What about these telescopic driving glasses I have heard of?" Tiny bioptic telescopes set into ordinary eyeglasses have been available for years. It is legal in about thirty states to drive with such devices, although there are additional visual acuity requirements for doing so.

Learning to use the telescopic lens is not easy. The small telescope is usually set into the spectacle lens of the better eye, slightly above the pupil line, and is used for spotting. A quick glance through the telescope verifies that the light is green, that the cross street is Maple, or that this is the "Cash-only" toll line. The driver then resumes looking through the center of the glasses, below the telescope, in order to continue ahead. This process requires practice with a trainer, and it usually takes several weeks or months to become proficient in it.

These driving lenses are still controversial among rehabilitation specialists. Some are very doubtful about their safety, while others believe that selective, well-trained people can drive safely with them. I feel that the patient with age-related macular degeneration, who is usually over sixty-five years old, is also likely to be developing problems with less rapid reflex time and diminished hearing. This would add to the danger involved in the use of these telescopic devices, which further narrow the field of vision. In my opinion, bioptic telescopes should be used only by younger people with low-vision problems caused by conditions other than age-related macular degeneration.

Making the Decision

So how should you make the decision about when to stop driving? For my patients, I now suggest that the decision process begin with a family consultation. You should have at hand your exact recent visual acuity measurements and your state's vision requirements for driving. A quiet, compassionate discussion should follow, with ample time for you to express your needs for driving and your emotional distress surrounding the issue. You should feel free to state your honest assessment of your driving ability, and you should listen respectfully to your loved ones' honest assessment of your ability.

You should also be aware that many states issue restricted driving licenses. These licenses generally restrict your driving to daylight hours and/or to certain locations. You and your family may then wish to conduct your own driving test by observing, on quiet streets, your ability to park, turn at specific locations, and avoid obstacles. If you meet the legal requirements for a restricted license and your ability to get to desired destinations appears intact, you should continue to drive.

But when the time comes for you to decide to end your driving, I hope you will take comfort from this thought. In our society, beginning to drive is associated with independence and maturity. However, when you voluntarily give up driving to ensure the safety of yourself, your passengers, and others unknown to you, the step you are taking is a testament to your wisdom and maturity.

My Own Story

At this point it is appropriate and important to bring my personal story up to date. It was on Independence Day, 2003, that I knew I would face my own *loss* of independence. I experienced the sudden blur, a dense hazy spot right in the center of vision in my "good" right eye. I knew immediately that a tiny blood vessel had burst in the center of my macular. Photo-dynamic therapy (PDT), which was then the best available treatment, stabilized my vision but left me with acuity below the level needed for a driving license in New York State, where I live.

I went through the process of denial that I'm sure occurs with most everyone who reaches this stage of AMD. I told myself that I could still see cars and traffic lights ahead of me, suppressing the fact that I well knew it was only by eccentric or off-center viewing that I could do this.

Fortunately for me and the pedestrians and drivers in my community, I quickly recognized the possibly fatal flaw in my thinking and turned in my still valid driver's license for a non-driver's photo ID.

This blow to my very sense of manhood, self-reliance, and independence was moderated to some degree for me by my devoted wife, an excellent driver, who was more than willing to chauffeur me around.

It is easy to understand the devastating feelings of someone without such an understanding spouse. However it is still critical for all of us to understand the danger of driving at 20, 30 or 50 miles per hour with a central blind spot obscuring part or all of another vehicle or person. We must consider all other options to function in a society increasingly dependent on the automobile. The possible solutions range from greater reliance on family, friends and neighbors to community organizations or governmental car service programs to paying taxi fares with the money saved on car maintenance and insurance. And there is the most healthful alternative: walking! Of course, those with a moderately severe visual impairment should take extra precaution in crossing streets, even, if necessary, carrying a small pocket telescope to scan the traffic.

In summary, giving up driving can be one of the most agonizing decisions to be made by people with AMD. For their own health and the safety of others, the decision must be faced squarely and honestly.

State Vision and Driving Requirements

Minimum acuity readings for restricted licenses

Alabama	20/60	Montana	20/50*
Alaska	20/100*	Nebraska	20/70
Arizona	20/60*	Nevada	20/60
California	---	New Jersey	---
Colorado	---	New Mexico	20/80
Connecticut	20/70*	New York	20/70*
Delaware	20/50	North Carolina	20/70*
D.C.	20/70*	North Dakota	20/60
Florida	---	Ohio	20/60
Hawaii	---	Oklahoma	20/100
Georgia	20/60*	Oregon	20/70
Idaho	20/40*	Pennsylvania	20/70*
Illinois	20/70	Rhode Island	---
Indiana	20/70	South Carolina	20/70*
Iowa	20/50	South Dakota	20/60
Kansas	20/60	Tennessee	20/60
Kentucky	20/60*	Texas	20/70*
Louisiana	20/70	Utah	20/70*
Maine	20/70	Vermont	---
Maryland	20/70	Virginia	20/70
Massachusetts	20/70	Washington	20/80*
Michigan	20/60	West Virginia	20/60*
Minnesota	20/70	Wisconsin	20/100*
Mississippi	20/70	Wyoming	20/100
Missouri	20/160*		

* Plus additional requirements
Note: An absence of a listed minimum requirement does not mean the state does not grant restricted licenses. These states usually evaluate applicants on an individual basis.
Source: "Summary of Medical Advisory Board Practices." TransAnalytics, LLC (June 2003).

CHAPTER 10

Special Tools, Special Help

Just because you have macular degeneration doesn't mean you have to give up all your favorite activities. With the help of a wide variety of low-vision aids and other tools, you can continue to read, pursue hobbies, enjoy the arts and sporting events, and maintain your independence. You can take and keep control of your life.

If you have just been recently diagnosed with macular degeneration or have a mild case, you may be functioning fairly well without low-vision aids. Or maybe you are finding it harder to read, sew, or do other close-up work but you've avoided addressing the issue out of embarrassment or simple lack of knowledge. The best advice I can give you—and the most important point of this entire chapter—is this: Don't wait another day before taking action.

There are two reasons for this. First, why deprive yourself of the joys of life if you don't have to? For instance, if you have always been a passionate reader but are reading less frequently now because of your low vision, there are tools and techniques you can use immediately to make reading more comfortable and pleasurable. (You can start right now with a simple step that will make it easier to read the rest of this book. Replace the bulb in the lamp you are using with one of higher wattage; 75 watts would be good, and 100 watts would be even better. More on the benefits of light in a moment.)

The other reason to take action on your low vision sooner rather than later is that it is much easier for a low-vision professional to evaluate your needs and demonstrate the use of various aids while your vision is still relatively good. For now, you may only need a good magnifying glass. However, with further visual loss always a possibility, you'll find it much easier over the long run to make a series of small incremental adjustments rather than wait and eventually be faced with the painful need to make a sudden and dramatic lifestyle change to accommodate your diminished vision.

This advice, to address the issue of your diminished vision sooner rather than later, frequently takes patients with early macular degeneration by surprise. "But my eye doctor didn't tell me to see a low-vision specialist" is a common response. Indeed, ophthalmologists typically don't automatically refer new macular degeneration patients to low-vision specialists. That is a mistake, albeit a well-intentioned one. Many ophthalmologists decide not to refer early-stage AMD patients to a low-vision specialist because they fear making their patients anxious about loss of vision. Ironically, an initial visit to a low-vision specialist is an excellent first step to relieving anxiety about vision loss.

Working with a Low-Vision Specialist

The process of addressing your diminished vision is called visual rehabilitation. The first step is a visit to a low-vision specialist. These are usually optometrists, and sometimes ophthalmologists, who specialize in low vision.

The best way to find a low-vision specialist is by asking your ophthalmologist for a referral. Your managed care plan may also be able to refer you to a low-vision specialist in your area. There are low-vision clinics associated with some hospitals and at medical school ophthalmology departments, optometry schools, and agencies such as the Lighthouse International. Finally, you may also find optometrists who offer low-vision services in the yellow pages under "Optometrists." Or go online at the website of the American Academy of Ophthalmology (www.AAO.org) and search under "low vision rehabilitation."

Unfortunately, the field of visual rehabilitation is relatively small. You may not have many possibilities for a provider, especially if you don't live in a metropolitan area. Ideally, though, here is what to look for in a low-vision center. The office has a quiet, soothing atmosphere with ample room for patients and their family members. It is well equipped with all the necessary technology to perform a complete eye examination. There are a wide range of low-vision aids available. The team leader is an ophthalmologist or optometrist, often aided by an ophthalmic assistant. The ophthalmologist or optometrist has access to an occupational therapist, a social worker, and a psychiatrist/psychologist.

Beginning Your Visual Rehabilitation

Now that we have set the stage, let me detail what you should expect, even ask for, in such a setting. The most important element is time. At least one hour is necessary to perform basic examinations and obtain a complete visual, social, and psychological history. Another thirty to sixty minutes, either during the same visit or in a subsequent one, is essential to discuss specific devices, techniques, and other possible therapeutic or preventive measures.

Your first visit should begin with a careful interview. You should prepare yourself to respond to a compassionate inquiry along the following lines:

1. What is the main difficulty with your vision—the one problem that you would like to be helped with most?

2. How have you fared with simple optical aids such as magnifiers?

3. How well do you manage the activities of daily living, such as shopping, cooking, cleaning, reading mail, writing checks and computer use?

4. How well do you understand what is wrong with your eyes?

5. What support system do you have: spouse, friends, siblings, other relatives or companion?

6. What are your feelings about the possibility of further visual loss, and the potential loss of independence, mobility, and recreation?

After the interview, the doctor should do a complete refraction so he or she can precisely measure your vision. This will allow him or her to identify the exact prescription of glasses that will provide the best possible visual acuity in each eye for both distance and near vision. This sounds like a rudimentary examination that should have been done earlier as a matter of course. Unfortunately, many patients with low vision frequently do not get this fine tuning, which often is of great help and can actually improve their vision.

Another part of your initial consultation with a low-vision specialist should be an exam that measures defects in the field of vision. This can often point to ways to work around the scotomas, or cloudy blind spots, caused by macular degeneration.

Finally, a good low-vision consultation should address the following additional services:

• Psychological counseling.

• Orientation and mobility training (O-and-M). This would involve everything from simple tips about care in walking to an actual referral to an O-and-M trainer.

• Audiological (hearing) evaluation.

• Occupational therapy and household management. This could involve helpful suggestions or even referral to an occupational therapy agency that could send trained personnel into your home for periods of specific on-site training.

• Community resources such as macular degeneration support groups and local state or federal offices that may offer services or programs.

• Discussions with you and your family members to ease any possible intrafamily tension resulting from your condition. The exact nature of the disability must be explained to everyone in the household so as to clear up any misunderstandings.

In addition to conducting the vision exam, taking your history, and providing the services just described, the low-vision specialist should discuss the best aids or devices to improve your functional vision. There are three general classes of devices available, and alone or in combination they can actually improve the visual performance of almost everyone with low vision.

Optical Aids

The most commonly used devices are called optical aids. These all consist of different arrangements of lenses that magnify the images presented to the retina. The principle of magnification is simple. If the image that is focused on the macula is large enough, it may be recognized even though patches may be missing due to the macula's degeneration.

Optical aids are available in the following forms:

Spectacle magnifiers with prisms. These devices are essentially super-high-powered reading glasses that allow you the use of both eyes while keeping your hands free. They are less obtrusive than some other low-vision devices, but they require that reading material be held six inches or less from your eyes.

Hand magnifiers. These vary in quality from those you buy in the drugstore to high quality, distortion-free instruments. They are very useful for spot tasks such as looking up telephone numbers, checking stock listings, and consulting a map. Everyone with low vision should have several, including one for the car and one that can be carried easily in a purse or pocket. One often-forgotten direction to patients is that if you wear bifocals, view an image with a magnifying glass through the distance, or top, portion of your eyeglasses, not through the reading, or bottom, section.

Stand magnifiers, which are used mainly for reading books. These are simply a form of hand magnifier attached to small legs or other supports so that they ride along the page at a proper, fixed distance. They are not very portable, and it does take practice to adjust to the smaller field of vision and the constant movement needed to keep the magnifier in place. However, they can be fitted with their own illumination system and can make for quite comfortable reading. Another note if you use bifocals: you will get best results from stand magnifiers by looking through them with the *reading* section of your glasses.

Loupes. These are small magnifying lenses that are held close to the eye, worn on the head, or attached to an existing eyeglass lens or frame. They are lightweight and can be used in very high powers for detailed examination of objects. However, they have a very small field of view.

Small telescopes. These are simply more complex optical systems wherein two lenses are at a fixed distance from each other within a tube. They are usually handheld to view or spot a distant object for a short period of time. Unfortunately, the field of view through the tube is quite small, and less light enters the tube, thereby making telescopes particularly difficult to use at night. A binocular spectacle-type telescope that offers a wider field of vision is also available.

Bioptics. These are miniaturized telescopes that are attached to your glasses slightly above the point behind which the pupil is aligned. They enable the user to simply lower the chin to "spot" through the telescopes, then raise the head to get a fuller field view through the glasses. There are new bioptic devices available with an auto-focus feature. When you are looking at an object through the device, the focus automatically changes so that objects at any distance can be seen more clearly.

Telemicroscopes. These are bioptics focused for close range. Usually only one is placed on a spectacle lens, just below the alignment point with the pupil. This position enables the device to act similarly to a bifocal lens, so that reading material can be held at a normal distance. Again, though, the field of view is smaller.

Nonoptical Aids

The second major category of low vision aids are referred to as nonoptical aids. This category includes anything else that makes visual and other routine tasks easier for the person with age-related macular degeneration or low vision of any other type-

Light. The single most important nonoptical visual aid is also the most readily available: increased light. Increasing the amount of light available will make reading more comfortable by heightening the contrast between the black letters on a page and the white paper. It also serves the function of "blasting through" the partial scotoma, or blind spot, of most people with AMD. The scotoma in the center of your vision is more like translucent waxed paper than opaque black paper. Intense light can more effectively penetrate this "waxed paper blur" to reach the still-functioning cells of the macula, and thereby give greater clarity to an image.

Two light sources are particularly helpful. A type of lightbulb named Chromalux, and another by General Electric called Enrich, both use a wavelength of light different from that of the traditional lightbulb, closer to that of sunlight, to increase the contrast between shades and thereby make the edges of letters sharper. I strongly recommend that all my patients place a 100-watt Enrich or Chromalux bulb in an adjustable, swivel-jointed (architect style) lamp for every visual task area. To keep the light from shining into your eye, the lamp must be placed so that it is in front of and slightly to the side of your head. I have also recently found another bulb type to fit into such a lamp, a miniature halogen floodlight of 45 watts. This produces a very bright white light, which helps to increase contrast sensitivity, making it easier to read print of poor quality.

Reading stands. Another underused nonoptical aid is an adjustable reading stand. When any form of magnification is used, the reading material and the eye must be kept at a fixed distance from each other.

This is most easily accomplished by placing your reading material on a stand like the Easy Reader or the Able Table, which will hold it at the proper angle and distance.

Absorptive filters. Usually likened to sunglasses, these can be effective both as preventive therapy and to increase contrast. Ultraviolet and blue light wavelengths may be particularly damaging to the lens of the eye and to the macula. I advise my patients to always protect their eyes from sunlight. Since ultraviolet radiation also penetrates the atmosphere even on hazy days, start a habit of wearing absorptive lenses in all daylight hours while out-of-doors. Almost all sunglasses available now will absorb over 95 percent of UVB, or ultraviolet B wavelength, the particularly damaging form. Specific wavelength-absorptive lenses of varying colors seem to help patients with age-related macular degeneration see slightly better. It may be useful to test the range from yellow to lavender to determine which is more effective for you. I find light to medium plum-colored lenses to be most helpful.

Reading and writing enhancers. Many devices are very useful in making reading and writing tasks easier. Some people may need nothing more than readily available large-print reading material, along with Enrich or Chromalux bulb lighting. Also useful are line isolators, called typoscopes, which are very inexpensive. They consist of black sheets of non-reflective material from which rectangular sections have been cut out to conform to the shape of a check or lines on a page to enable writing on stationery. Typoscopes often make daily life easier on a routine basis. Finally, simple black felt-tipped pens are best for writing anything because of their increased contrast on white paper.

Useful gadgets, hints, and services. There are many household appliances that can make daily life easier for people with low vision, such as talking watches and calculators and cooking appliances that use sounds to indicate when a roast is done or when a cup is filled with fluid.

There are also many games and hobbies specially designed for people with low vision. If you use a computer, you can set your software to display text, icons, and toolbars in an enlarged typeface. (Quick tip: While on the Internet, you can quickly enlarge the size of the text on most web pages by depressing the Control key and + key simultaneously.) In addition, there are various free and low-cost services available to people with low vision, from access to free information calls from telephone companies to free large-print magazine delivery. Please check Resources for a comprehensive list of services, supplies, and catalogues of many nonoptical aids.

High-Tech Devices

We now come to the third major category of low-vision devices, namely electronic and high-tech aids. Great advances are being made rapidly in the technology of helping visually impaired people see better. The basic tool is the closed circuit television, or CCTV. The principle is that a small video camera transmits the image of anything it is pointed at to a television screen, where the image is displayed in an enlarged format. Some units are all self-contained, while others use your TV screen. The degree of magnification can be very great, and good color transmission even allows the viewing of photographs, which would not otherwise be discernible. Of special note is the new Amazon Kindle, an e-book reader. The Kindle's easy-to-read text can be enlarged to a comfortable size, and can even read passages of text aloud in an automated voice. Prices of these high-tech reading devices range between $350 and $3,000.

For individuals with a more severe visual handicap, voice synthesizers can be useful. These text-to-voice devices have improved dramatically in recent years. If you simply place a printed page or a book into one of these newer models, a pleasant voice will read the material back to the listener. There is even computer software that can read your documents and e-mail to you. The best advice is to acquire catalogues from some of the companies that specialize in these kinds of devices; several are listed in Resources.

Super-miniaturized video cameras mounted on headgear or large spectacle-like devices are one area of emerging technology that holds great promise in the low-vision field. The cameras present an image on tiny screens in front of the viewer's eyes, so that magnification of surroundings can be viewed at any distance. A prototype of this device, in which the tiny cameras and visual screens were located in a helmet, showed promise but wasn't successful in the market because of its appearance and weight. A similar device that looks like a large pair of eyeglasses is now available. But instead of looking through the glasses, the user focuses on images projected onto tiny video screens mounted inside the device just in front of the eyes.

Such vision aids will likely evolve into highly useful tools for many macular degeneration patients. Although they may be costly and difficult to acquire at first, it is likely that—as with most technology—they will become readily available at moderate costs within several years of their introduction.

Tools I Use

I subscribe to the maxim that there is no single-purpose visual aid for low vision. I use a variety of aids and techniques, each for a specific purpose.

• I have changed the bulbs in my desk lamp, in my bedside lamp, and wherever else I read or write to a 100-watt GE Enrich bulb or a 45-watt halogen miniature flood bulb.

• I always carry a high-quality, 3-X or 5-X pocket magnifier from Bausch & Lomb, which has a slide-out lens in a plastic case. This is very handy for prices and menus, especially when it is used with the small, high-powered penlight I keep in my pocket.

• I also keep with me an Eschenbach 6-X monocular telescope, a small device that can be used for both distance and close-up magnification. I use it for spotting street and store signs and for quickly spot-checking faces.

• A personal favorite of mine for the theater and spectator sports is the Beecher Mirage Telescopic Spectacles. These offer 4-X to 8-X power and provide a relatively wide field of vision. They are lightweight and look like a small pair of ordinary binoculars mounted in a traditional eyeglass frame. They allow me to see a large portion of a stage or ball-field, and they don't look particularly conspicuous. I also use spectacle-binoculars called Max TV, which provides a 2-X magnification that is very suitable for TV or movies.

Of course, items that I find useful may not be the best devices for others. Ultimately, there is no substitute for working with a well-trained, low-vision specialist.

Contrast Sensitivity

The measurement of a visual function called contrast sensitivity is rather time consuming and therefore often neglected by most eye-care professionals. Contrast sensitivity refers to the ability of the normal retinal rod and cone cells to distinguish minute differences in shades of gray, such as a gradation from white to black. There are methods by which the retina can be evaluated by determining the smallest difference in shading that can be detected. This ability of the retina decreases early in the onset of AMD and progresses at a rapid rate. Thus poor contrast sensitivity complicates reading ability, night driving, and bright light adaptation even *before* severe vision changes. This problem can be helped a great deal by increasing the amount of light falling on a page or object so that type or the object is more discernible.

CHAPTER 11

Adapting Your Home for Easier Living

In spite of everything that your family and friends can do to provide help and support, you may find the tasks of daily living obstacles to a happy, fulfilling life. However, with a little thought and planning, you can make modest changes in your home that will yield great benefits in your daily life. Here are some practical and easy recommendations, some of which have been adapted from a useful small volume from the American Foundation for the Blind entitled *Making Life More Livable* by Irving R. Dickman.

Start with a room-by-room walk-through of your home. Do this with someone who can help you make any necessary changes.

Light, Light, Light!

For people with age-related macular degeneration, the key to improvement is lighting, and incandescent rather than fluorescent. Fluorescent lights, typically found in kitchens and bathrooms and increasingly in table lamps and ceiling fixtures, emit a bluish light that frequently flickers. Incandescent lights are better because they are closer to the wavelength of sunlight; they provide softer, higher-contrast illumination than fluorescent lights. (Enrich or Chromalux brand bulbs are particularly helpful.) Also, the higher the wattage the better. Older people with age-related macular degeneration often struggle with a few 60-watt bulbs all over the house. It is far better to have many areas of 100-watt focused lighting or new fluorescent bulbs.

One possible problem with increased lighting is glare, particularly for the elderly, whose pupils do not constrict adequately to cut down excessive light. During your walk-through watch for glare spots or slippery areas on hardwood floors or linoleum. In such cases, nonslip carpeting or runners may be useful.

In the Kitchen

• Many kitchens have adequate overall lighting but insufficient spot lighting. A small, portable architect-type, triple-jointed lamp is very useful to have on a counter to be moved wherever needed.

• If you find it hard to identify the contents of jars and cans, relabel them with peel-and-stick labels using a broad-tipped black felt pen.

• Tactile markers are wonderfully useful to help you identify stove or refrigerator settings; they also enable you to differentiate the regular from the decaffeinated coffee can, for example, or assist you in any other separation process that can be helped by the sense of touch. "Touch dots" come in raised colors from an eighth of an inch to three-eighths of an inch in diameter, and they self-stick anywhere. For instance, if you place one on the off point on the stove dials and others at the high, medium, and low settings, setting and adjusting your burners and oven can be a snap.

• Use gadgets. Catalogues such as those of the LS&S Group (800-468-4789; www.lssgroup.com) or of Low-Vision.com (800-826-4200; www.lowvision.com) have lots of useful items, ranging from simple kitchen helpers to sophisticated electronic devices. For example, the Magna Wonder Knife can be set to slice bread or meat at a predetermined thickness. Such items are particularly useful when used on white cutting boards to provide high contrast. There are also measuring spoons set by clicks, easily set timers, and thermometers that say the temperature.

The Bedroom

Bedrooms are the site of many household accidents.

The hazards are increased with decreased vision, poor lighting, and the need to get out of bed at night while fatigued or stiff.

• Lighting. Always use a night-light, which helps reduce the adjustment time for your eyes when a brighter light is turned on. A dimmer switch on your bedside lamp can make it easier to turn the light on and off and will help you avoid the difficult adjustment to a sudden bright light. Use additional light sources to illuminate drawers, shelves, and closets. Finding the proper color socks in the drawer is made much easier by having a bright lamp nearby or even a large flashlight. Remember, lighting helps break through scotomas!

• Keep the path through the center of the room and to the bathroom clear. In dimmer light, the central scotoma of your macular degeneration will obscure even relatively large objects. Push furniture next to the walls and keep doors open. Be particularly aware of protruding footboards on beds, which are frequently the cause of painful injuries.

• Practice efficiency by organizing your life and surroundings. In the bedroom, for example, put your socks in one part of the drawer, underwear in another. Use trays for small items on the bureau. Organize your closet by color or style.

The Bathroom

Another obvious danger zone is the bathroom. Hard, slippery floors, projecting edges, and glare add to ordinary difficulties.

• Slip protection can be provided by wall-to-wall quick-dry carpeting, grab bars on tubs and in the shower, and brightly colored nonskid mats or tape in the bathtub.

• Single-knob faucets with thermostatic settings are easier to use than traditional twin faucets. Using a liquid soap dispenser is much easier than finding a bar of soap.

• Shaving may be easier with an electric razor than a blade. An electric shaver can be used fairly effectively by feel alone; shaving with blades, on the other hand, requires far more visual acuity.

• Applying makeup can be made easier by using a magnifying mirror, particularly the type with built-in lighting.

• Talking bathroom scales are particularly useful, as is a talking oral thermometer for those times when you are ill. There are also prescription bottle magnifiers and talking blood pressure monitors.

Living Room

The living room is an area where loose carpeting or highly polished wooden floors can be a danger. Subdued lighting in living rooms and small end tables or low coffee tables may also present problems.

• Once again, lighting must be increased to help you function in the living room. Brighter and lighter walls and drapes are also useful.

• The use of nonskid waxes and double-sided sticky tape on all loose runners or carpets can prevent falls (in the case of normal-sighted people, as well!).

• For watching television, the simplest and least expensive maneuver is to move a comfortable chair within two or three feet of the set. This creates a magnification of proximity and enables most people with age-related macular degeneration to enjoy their favorite programs. Television-enlarging screens are inexpensive and may be very helpful. Those who do not want to sit so close to the TV can also use simple telescopic devices.

• Gadgetry in the living room involves mostly dimmer switches to vary illumination for mood lighting for visitors to very bright, non-glare lighting for your own use. Recreational games of many types from playing cards to checkers and Scrabble are available in enlarged formats from organizations such as LS&S or LowVision.com.

Hallways and Stairs

Steps and stairs present a real challenge to people with AMD because the normal impulse to focus on the exact location of the step's edge gives erroneous information. Most falls occur when one is descending the stairs or stepping down from the curb, because the leading edge of the step may not be visible against the flat surface of the next step.

• Lighting, of course, should be increased in all areas where there are steps. In addition, use luminescent switchplates in hallways, which are often difficult to light well. To highlight switchplates in dim areas try applying brightly colored tape around them.

• Yellow or orange reflective tape placed along the leading edge of the steps can help you distinguish one step from the next. If a double or triple width of tape is placed on the topmost and the bottommost step, it may add extra certainty.

• Guide rails in the hallway near the stairs and bright-colored handrails alongside the stairs are also helpful.

Out-of-Doors

There is absolutely no reason for anyone with age-related macular degeneration to be housebound, and I strongly urge all my patients to make every effort to maintain normal social contacts and duties outside the home. This not only builds self-confidence and independence, but also helps avoid the depression brought on by isolation. There are, however, a few specialized needs that can be addressed.

• Keys may not be easy to tell apart. Locking and unlocking doors, mailboxes, and the like can be made easier if you use keys in different colors or shapes. Most hardware stores sell plastic key rings that can be used to differentiate one key from another.

• Elevators present particular problems, both in finding the correct button to push and in keeping track of which floor to get off. The simplest step to take also demonstrates your acceptance of the disability, a major advance toward new freedoms. If someone is in the elevator, ask him or her to press the button for your floor and then ask to be notified when that floor has been reached. Another alternative involves the use of the pocket magnifier and pocket telescope. The magnifier would usually allow the number to be seen on the buttons, and the telescope can be used to spot the number of the floor arrived at.

• Supermarkets are the source of many problems because of the dizzying array of choices and prices and the abundance of people and carts. Choose a time of day to shop when the store is least crowded. You might also find it useful to use technology aids. At the supermarket shelves, a magnifying loupe temporarily attached to your eyeglasses is useful for reading labels and prices. The lighting in supermarkets poses further problems. There is usually too much overhead fluorescent lighting, which produces glare, and too little lighting at the shelf level. Carry a pocket flashlight to illuminate the item being examined with a magnifying loupe. Until such time as stores install better lighting and more readable packaging, shopping is going to consume more time, require more effort, and be more frustrating than it was before you had AMD.

So which of these suggestions should you take? Frankly, most macular degeneration patients will not need to adopt all of them. Each of us reacts differently to our visual disability, and we all have our own individual needs. However, if the simple changes outlined in this chapter can make your life easier and less stressful, don't hesitate to implement them!

CHAPTER 12

Issues for Caregivers

This chapter is for the caregivers: the spouse, siblings, children, grandchildren, companions and friends of the person with age-related macular degeneration. You are faced with three issues. First, you must understand the nature of your loved one's disability. Second, you must learn how best to react to this new development in the life of your loved one and how to help most effectively. And third, you must take particular care to help him or her avoid a state of prolonged and disabling depression that can often evolve from low vision.

Macular degeneration patients are perpetually plagued by the scotoma, or central blind spot, that is the hallmark of AMD. A normal-sighted person finds it really hard to imagine the frustration of not being able to see exactly what you want to look at. Life with AMD means not being able to look through, around, over, or under this "damned spot" that constantly follows your every eye movement and blurs out a varying amount of whatever you try to see.

The closest anyone with normal vision can get to

evaluating the sensation would be to place a circle of opaque Scotch tape, three quarters of an inch in diameter, directly in the center of each lens in a pair of eyeglasses. Then, while you are keeping your eyes locked in a straight-ahead position, move your head and try to look at objects. You can never see the targeted object directly; instead, you see only other things that are out of sharp focus with the periphery of your vision. The problem would be enormously worsened by having the tape move wherever you move your eyes. Even with this image of how an AMD patient sees, you will still find it hard to understand the exact nature of your loved one's disability, because the nature of the visual disability varies widely from patient to patient.

Of course, caregivers vary in their responses to their loved one's condition. We can divide the responses that family members and friends typically have toward the visually impaired person's needs into three categories: the overprotectors, the deniers, and the acceptance/adjusters.

Overprotectors

The overprotectors are often those who, with the best of intentions, can still undermine the patient's sense of independence and self-esteem. Finding a balance between helping and taking over is not always easy.

Remember that your parent or grandparent still can and must maintain his or her own life. Resist the temptation to take over all routine tasks when you visit. After all, when you are not with your loved one, he or she is managing without you. By rushing in to provide assistance when it's not needed, you risk fostering resentment or a sense of futility on the part of your relative. If you see your loved one having some difficulty with a task, ask casually if you can help. If your offer is declined, don't pursue the issue. And now a note to the AMD patient: Be honest about when you need help and when you don't. Ask for it when you need it and decline the offer of it when you don't. If you are honest about your needs, you will maximize both your independence and your ease of living, and you won't frustrate your friends and relatives.

Deniers

If the family denies that anything is happening at all, this may be even more destructive of the patient's self-image and integrity than overprotection. People with age-related macular degeneration do not suddenly appear different, nor do they often act differently than when their sight was normal. The patient tries to appear self-sufficient and to prove to everyone that things are really not so bad.

Nevertheless, you may notice that household

chores are neglected, financial matters are not dealt with, and regular meals are neglected. You must not deny that anything is amiss, even if your spouse or parent does certain things easily, such as find a chair to sit in or pick up a fork properly. The insidious effect that this negative attitude will have on the patient is to inhibit his or her ability to ask for help when it is really needed.

And now some words to the patient about how denial on your part can have a bad effect on your family and friends. A macular degeneration patient who allows pride to keep him or her from being open about the handicap risks many problems. Greater care and more time may be needed with stairs and curbs, and it may be very important to use a large-print deck of cards for playing bridge. If these issues are not openly discussed, people may judge you to be clumsy, unfriendly, or unintelligent. Again, the best advice is to be completely open with everyone—relatives, friends and even new acquaintances—about your disability and your need for help or special accommodations.

Accepting/Adjusting Families

The accepting/adjusting family can do the most good in practical and emotional—and even, possibly, physiological—terms. By displaying patience, hopefulness, and encouragement, and by offering support only when it is needed, these compassionate families may actually be providing valuable therapy for the AMD patient.

This phenomenon has recently been demonstrated in a review of the physiology of expectancy. A large part of the efficacy of drugs, even ones that have no active ingredients (placebos), is due to special receptors in the brain. These centers interpret the feelings of expected results and send signals to the target organ effectuating at least part of the improvement. This effect has been demonstrated to show positive results in such diverse conditions as arthritis, asthma, and growing hair on balding spots.

Since the biochemistry of vision is so complex and is tied intimately to brain cells, a hopeful and positive attitude—along with the antioxidant nutritional therapy described in chapter 7—may actually stabilize or improve functional vision in those whose maculas are not severely damaged.

How to Help

Deciding where, when, and how to offer help, and when to withhold it, is hard. Certainly, you can start by helping the patient modify his or her home in small but useful ways that will serve to enhance independence and self-esteem. (See chapter 11 for specific suggestions.) However, you should be aware that taking even small steps to accommodate your loved one's loss of vision may call his or her attention to the reality of the need for help and thus make him or her sad or depressed for a while.

It is not necessarily safe to wait until the AMD patient asks for help. Denial and the irrational fear of impending blindness may be so great that the patient may not act in time to avoid harmful accidents.

Nowhere is the issue of safety more important than with driving. At some point in the progression of the disease, your loved one will almost certainly need to stop driving, probably first at night and in inclement weather, and then completely. (For guidelines on driving, see chapter 9.) However, most AMD patients are reluctant to curtail their driving because of the associated loss of independence. The burden of suggesting and perhaps ultimately imposing restrictions on driving often falls on caregivers. You must be vigilant about your loved one's driving ability. If you are concerned, you should suggest an eye exam to ascertain whether the patient meets the legal vision requirements for driving. If such a suggestion meets resistance, as it sometimes does, you may need to take the difficult step of refusing to drive with the AMD patient until he or she takes the eye exam. As difficult as this issue may be to address, it is a matter of life and death for your loved one, you, and others on the road.

Provide Encouragement
But Not False Hope

However many times the doctor explains the basic condition to the patient, the exact nature of macular degeneration seems difficult for many people to grasp. As a caregiver, you must encourage your loved one without offering false hope. Reassure your loved one again and again that he or she will not go blind. Emphasize over and over that the condition was not brought on by some dereliction on the patient's part. Excessive reading, too little light, or too much television are *not* causes of macular degeneration.

Reassure your spouse or parent of your own understanding of the nature of his or her disability. For instance, say that you are aware that he or she can pick up a quarter from the rug but still cannot turn the oven on properly. Even small physical limitations may engender fear and anxiety levels that are very high. Offer observations and suggestions that may help your loved one cope effectively in his or her low-vision environment.

Your loved one may, for example, inadvertently acquire a negative social habit as he or she learns to use eccentric fixation to see around the central blind spot. With eccentric fixation you must focus the eyes on a point *slightly away* from the target object in order to see it more clearly. When the target is the face of another person, as it is in a conversation, your loved one's companions may feel that he or she is not paying attention to what they are saying. As much as we try to understand such a need, it can be distancing to never have eye contact in a conversation. Gently point out to your loved one that if he or she intermittently looks directly into the blurred area that is the face of the person opposite, it will give that person a sense of greater connection in the conversation. This is especially important in dealing with children, who are more likely to misinterpret the look of eccentric fixation as a lack of interest.

Strange Sightings

Your spouse or parent with age-related macular degeneration may be experiencing a disturbing but insignificant mild hallucination often connected to visual impairment. In 1760, Dr. Charles Bonnet published the first report of a visually impaired person who reported seeing a perfectly formed phantom object. What has since been called the Charles Bonnet syndrome is still neither well understood nor widely recognized by most physicians. Yet this syndrome is remarkably common in people with a visual loss, particularly in cases of AMD.

The condition is so disturbing to many people that they will not mention it, especially to friends and family members, out of a fear that they will be labeled crazy or senile. The experience can be quite disorienting, since it occurs when the person is fully alert, eyes wide open. Suddenly an image appears, without any apparent cause and totally outside of the patient's control. The hallucination, which is usually in color, may be of a specific object, such as a flower or an animal, or it may be a brief series of changing designs. The images almost never move, and the vision is usually present for just a few seconds and then suddenly disappears. During and after the episode, most people are quite aware that the image is a hallucination and that it does not exist.

Recent studies have shown that almost 20 percent of patients with age-related macular degeneration have experienced this symptom, and those with worse vision experience the phenomenon more frequently than those with better vision. Interestingly, only about a third of these people admitted having the experience without at first being specifically asked about it and then being reassured that it was a common occurrence with no psychiatric significance. Patients then greeted this news with more detailed descriptions of what they "saw," usually to the surprise of family members present.

There is no known scientific basis to explain the phenomenon, but it is known that in patients undergoing laser surgery to the macula, approximately 45 percent will report seeing twinkling or colored lights within hours or a day of the laser treatment. What is not widely recognized, probably because of patient reluctance to admit it, is that about 15 percent of people undergoing laser treatment will see the hallucinations associated with Charles Bonnet syndrome. No one should worry about this. There is absolutely no connection between this syndrome and mental illness of any kind. And for those who have had or are considering laser surgery, please be assured that the lights or visions do *not* indicate that the laser treatment has caused permanent damage.

Some people with age-related macular degeneration become suspicious and mistrustful of others. This is a personality trait that, unfortunately, is common among patients with severe AMD, especially as they age. Unable to check the actions and facial expressions of those around them, people with dramatic vision loss can begin to feel isolated and mistrustful. This can accentuate any tendency to blame others and in some cases can lead to sad, unwarranted terminations of close relationships.

Watch for Signs of Depression

Finally, as a caregiver for a person with AMD, you must look for signs of depression. The association between aging, vision loss, and depression is often unrecognized by family, friends, and even most eye doctors, who should know better.

Depression and illness or disability are often connected. Disabilities can and do lead to normal or abnormal levels of depression. In fact, depression itself results in greater degrees of illness and functional disability. Although not everyone with age-related macular degeneration develops clinical depression, recent evidence indicates that close to 40 percent of visually impaired elderly people develop significant depressive symptoms within a year of the diagnosis. In equivalent groups of normal-sighted people, the figure averages about 20 percent.

What is an equally significant finding for caregivers is that the severity of the visual loss is *not* what correlates to depression. Instead, the depression appears to be directly related to three factors, all of which may be mitigated by knowledgeable caregivers. The first is the patient's own self-perceived state of his or her general health and visual function. The second is the presence or absence of a network of close emotional ties with family and friends. The third factor is the understandable but destructive response by the patient of anger and blaming others.

Respond to misperceptions on the part of the patient about his or her state of health by offering explanatory information. Emphasize your loved one's residual visual capability and provide repeated assurances that he or she will not go totally blind. Maintain or build a strong family and social network, for it is critically important that your loved one feel, and be, part of a broader community. Relatives and friends must repeatedly demonstrate the solidity of the emotional bonds that link you together. The third predictor of depression, a tendency to anger and lay blame, is often handled better by a professional counselor.

Since the person visually handicapped with age-related macular degeneration will rarely be diagnosed as depressed by the attending ophthalmologist, family and friends must become aware of the signs of significant depression and must seek help if any of these symptoms appear:

• A loss of interest and/or pleasure in previously enjoyed activities

• A persistent mood of depression

• A decrease in appetite and weight

• An inability to sleep or a tendency to sleep too much

• Listlessness or fatigue

• Feelings of worthlessness or guilt

- Episodes of unexplained agitation

- An inability to concentrate for even short periods of time

- Recurrent thoughts of death or suicide

One of the difficulties in the field of low-vision rehabilitation is that depression is often the basis for a patient's unwillingness to deal with the necessary program of aids and training. Some form of psychotherapy or psychopharmacology may be called for. In most cases, prolonged psychiatric care is not necessary. The newer, shorter cognitive approach is particularly useful, and one or another of the new psychoactive drugs can produce dramatic changes in the depressed state.

I can't emphasize enough the value of family and peer support as tools for preventing or alleviating depression among people with age-related macular degeneration. The loss of any degree of vision creates a stress syndrome that has long been known to result in a cascade of negative effects. These include not only emotional responses but also very measurable physiological changes ranging from hormones in the adrenal gland to chemical neurotransmitters in the brain. Social support can act as a buffer against some of these changes. Important examples of valuable social support include the simple reassurance that anxiety, frustration, depression, and even denial are quite normal responses to the situation. Reassure your loved one that these mechanisms can provide time to absorb the loss and can set the stage for the rehabilitative process. Take active steps to prevent the AMD patient from becoming isolated, a situation that often results from the decreased mobility and less frequent social intercourse that tends to occur with vision loss.

Another effective way to avoid isolation, which aggravates a sense of depression, is to help your loved one find and participate in macular degeneration support groups. Unfortunately, there are fewer support groups for macular degeneration patients than there are for many other diseases. Your eye doctor may be able to direct you to a local support group if one exists. If not, there is always the possibility of starting your own group by posting your intention on the Internet or in the receptionist's area of your ophthalmologist's office. Responses will undoubtedly be forthcoming. If you'd like to hook up with a support network over the Internet, start by searching for "macular degeneration support group." You'll find several organizations that offer online networking for people with AMD.

Unfortunately, most ophthalmologists do not refer their patients to support groups. Patients are often angry at their doctors for not having referred them to peer support groups. Many patients give credit to their groups for having turned their lives around. One statistic has revealed that on average as much as seven years will go by before someone with impaired vision is connected with a rehabilitation service. Please don't let your loved one wait nearly that long!

CHAPTER 13

The Eye of the Beholder

"A person's own toothache is always much worse than someone else's broken leg." That was often my father's response when, as a child, I would complain unduly about some annoying ache or pain. His attitude confused me, because I felt that this apparently unfeeling aphorism stood in sharp contrast to my father's kind and gentle nature.

As I became older and wiser, though, I realized that the remark was simply an acerbic insight into a frailty common to most of us: We allow our personal afflictions to obscure not just the suffering of others but also the path through or around our own self-pity.

The path from despair to repair is one that must be traveled alone by each of us. But perhaps by relating my own experience, along with those of several extraordinary people who contributed mightily to the world's visual pleasure despite their own loss of sight, I can provide support to those just starting on their own paths to personal renewal.

A Cascade of Feelings

My own journey began with a cascade of feelings that led, domino-like, to a deepening sense of despair. As I first began to appreciate the ramifications of my diagnosis, I was consumed by my impending losses: the ability to perform the demanding surgery I had found so rewarding, my enjoyment of reading and the arts, my independence, and, above all, the delight in seeing the beautiful faces of my wife, children, and grand-children.

Then I began to criticize myself for these feelings of self-pity and self-absorption, which I interpreted as evidence of a personal weakness or a character flaw. I became angry at myself for not rising to what I thought was the proper level of philosophical detach-ment from my fate, for failing to appreciate what my father would have pointed out: others were much worse off than I was.

I soon also found myself with an additional sense of oppression, one experienced by many people with age-related macular degeneration. The disease often starts in one eye but often involves the other at a later date. This waiting for the other shoe to drop turned out to be more upsetting than I had expected.

My primary scotoma, in my left eye, is shaped like a lima bean, and covers the exact center of my field of vision in that eye. The scotoma blurs and distorts the face and upper chest of someone standing six feet away from me; it completely obscures an object, such as a car, fifty feet away. Fortunately, while near normal vision remained in my good right eye, I could ignore the scotoma in my left. What I could not ignore was the dread of developing a blind spot in my right eye.

When that spot finally appeared, I reacted with a surprising mix of relief and horror. The scotoma that developed in my right eye is peanut-shaped and off-center, meaning that as a whole—at least as of this writing—I can still see. But when I close my right eye and look at the world through my more impaired left, I continue to experience the agonizing frustration of trying to see around "that damned spot." And with my left eye closed, I quickly slide into a feeling of dread associated with the constant awareness that some-day, perhaps soon, I will lose the vision that I still have in my right eye.

The feelings of frustration and fear never fully go away, but I now see that there is something to be said for the slow progression of this disease. It is really a kindness of sorts, for it gives one time to think, pre-pare, adjust, and remediate. This time is of great val-ue if it is used to one's advantage. In my case, it has enabled me to help my patients both from the outside, as a physician, and from the inside, as a fellow suffer-er. In the cases of most of the patients I have worked with, it has helped them transcend denial, despair, depression, and other emotions to emerge with a different lifestyle. I have found that the path to this new lifestyle is marked by a blending of the serenity of acceptance with the equanimity of a different kind of fulfillment.

While traveling this path myself, I drew strength and insight from the lives of several great artists whose sight became as frustratingly distorted or obscured as has my own. Claude Monet, the painter of those indescribably beautiful water lilies, lived with devastatingly advanced cataracts. Mary Cassatt, perhaps the greatest American impressionist, was tormented by cataracts and diabetic retinopathy. Camille Pissarro, called the father of French impressionism, struggled to work with his eyes often covered with pus from obstructed tear ducts. Edgar Degas, whose ballerinas and softly evocative scenes of dancers and bathers bring joy to so many all over the world, probably had a form of macular degeneration. Edvard Munch, the Norwegian artist perhaps best known for the haunting image in *The Scream,* furiously worked to "paint around" the ghostly blur of debris from floating blood clots that may have been a result of a macular hemorrhage. Finally, the American painter Georgia O'Keeffe, with her brilliant, often luminous large canvases of flowers and plants, suffered a loss of vision late in life from severe macular degeneration. The stories of these artists' struggles with their vision are dramatically related in a wonderful book, *The Eye of the Artist*, by two brilliant professors of ophthalmology, Dr. Michael Marmor in California and Dr. James Ravin in Ohio. Many of the following biographical details are drawn from their book.

Claude Monet

Claude Monet (1840-1926), whose early painting *Impressionism: Sunrise* gave that famous artistic movement its name, is renowned for his artistic depiction of light. His studies of haystacks, Rouen Cathedral, and of course, the water lilies in his own garden, provide evidence of an awe-inspiring prism-like ability to break down light into its fundamental color components. "Monet Refuses the Operation," by Lisel Mueller, the poem that appears at the beginning of this book, expresses beautifully and poignantly Monet's ability to transform deep emotions into artistic vision.

It is even more inspiring, then, to consider Monet's artistic ability in light of his years-long struggle with declining vision, first from a dense cataract in his right eye and then from one in his left. What Mueller's poem does not fully reveal is the torment and frustration that Monet endured as he tried to decide whether to gamble his remaining sight on a then-risky cataract operation. He was terrified by the prospect of surgery, especially after he saw the poor result of similar surgery in his artist friend Mary Cassatt.

In coming to terms with his loss of vision, Monet apparently experienced the intense frustration that so many people with age-related macular degeneration endure. "I stayed for hours under the harshest sun...forcing myself to...resume my interrupted task and recapture the freshness that had disappeared from my palette," he wrote in 1918. "Wasted efforts! What I painted was more and more dark, more and more like an old picture, and when the attempt was over, I compared it to former works. I would be seized by a frantic rage and slash all my canvases with my pen knife."

Monet ultimately underwent the surgery and suffered through a very difficult postoperative period for two years, but he did finally regain some of his "freshness" and continued painting to the day he died.

Mary Cassatt

The story of Mary Cassatt (1845-1926) may be instructive to AMD patients perplexed by claims of "dramatic new cures" for the disease. Although she never achieved the same level of fame as some of her contemporaries, Cassatt is now held by many to be one of America's foremost artists.

In addition to cataracts, Cassatt was unfortunate enough to also have diabetes, which itself can lead to severe eye problems. This was prior to the discovery of insulin, so her untreated diabetes probably complicated her cataract surgery, which resulted in further vision loss. Probably as a result of her diminished eyesight, her brilliant, crisp scenes of mothers and children were replaced by a coarser type of painting, harsher in color.

In an effort to treat her diabetes, and also possibly her cataracts, Cassatt underwent radium inhalation treatments. At the time, radium was widely considered as a harmless curative agent for a variety of ailments, even by many in the medical establishment. In 1920, *The American Journal of Ophthalmology* published an article by two well-regarded ophthalmologists who claimed that 84 percent of cataract patients treated with radium showed varying degrees of improvement. Another article in a prominent journal of radiology stated that the application of radium would be harmless to the eyes. It was not until many workers with radium developed severe problems that the real dangers of the element were recognized. (Marie Curie herself, the pioneer in radiation, developed cataracts, possibly due to her own exposure to radium.)

Cassatt's misadventure with a new, "harmless"

treatment underscores the need for caution in evaluating any of the dramatic claims of traditional or alternative medicine.

Camille Pissarro

Camille Pissarro's story shows us how, with determination and creativity, it is almost always possible to work around adversity. A leader of French impressionism with Monet, Pissarro (1830-1903) had a chronic blockage of the tear canal, which flows from a small opening at the inner corner of the lower eyelid into the nose. This canal normally drains tears into the nose and allows fresh tears, formed by the tear gland under the outer corner of the upper lid, to continually lubricate the eyeball with fresh, clean fluid. When the canal is obstructed, the tears stagnate, become infected, and form a thick, cloudy film over the cornea. Pissarro had to endure this condition for at least the last fifteen years of his life. (Today this problem can be corrected with surgery; when Pissarro developed the condition, in the late nineteenth century, there was no effective surgical treatment for it.)

Pissarro found that he had to avoid wind, dust, and bright lights, so he adapted his technique. He felt that keeping a bandage over the eye helped. He also found that since he was unable to work outdoors, he would paint indoors while looking outward. Some of his beautiful scenes of Paris are from that period.

Edgar Degas

Many are familiar with Edgar Degas's evocative works of ballerinas practicing, couples dancing, and women bathing. What is not as well known is that his progression into sculpture and the use of pastels, rather than the more intricate use of oils, was dictated by his diminishing eyesight. There are several conflicting opinions as to what caused his vision loss, but the most likely diagnosis appears to be a form of macular degeneration that can occur at a younger age. Degas (1834—1917) was only thirty-six when he began to have severe symptoms, and his vision deteriorated to the point of what would now be classified as legal blindness. The exact nature of what tormented him as an artist will be familiar to anyone with a central scotoma. His artist friend Walter Sickert reported that Degas described the blind spot in the center of his vision as a torment. Sickert wrote: "It was natural that during the years when I knew him, that he should sometimes have spoken of the torment that it was to draw when he could only see around the spot at which he was looking and never the spot itself."

Degas also had to deal with the lack of understanding so common among the friends and family of people with age-related macular degeneration. An art dealer wrote that "Degas used to pretend to be more blind than he was in order to not recognize people he wanted to avoid." As proof of this, the dealer stated that after complaining of his "poor eyes," Degas would take out his watch and say the time. The art dealer was obviously not aware that while details of a face or a painting would not be clear with a central scotoma, large black hands on the white face of a pocket watch would very likely be visible, especially if Degas had learned the technique of eccentric fixation to improve definition and clarity.

Edvard Munch

Edvard Munch (1863-1944) was a Norwegian artist who painted in the striking colors of impressionism, of which his most famous painting, *The Scream,* is an excellent example. He always had poor vision in his left eye, but at age sixty-seven he experienced a sudden gross distortion of vision in his right eye from a bleeding retinal artery or vein, an event that may have been related to a wet form of age-related macular degeneration. The diagnosis was never fully established, but we know that he must have had a gross and irregular scotoma because he incorporated its imagery into many of his paintings. A self-portrait in bed shows him covering his weak left eye with one hand and viewing a large black object at the foot of his bed, an object that has the toothy grin of a death's head painted at the lower end. This period of visual impairment lasted only a year and did not leave him permanently disabled. Munch reveals another instance where the eye gives us raw information that our minds and spirit can transform to whatever brilliant scenes our determination can forge.

Georgia O'Keeffe

Georgia O'Keeffe's experience with vision loss also offers lessons to modern-day AMD patients. She likely had a predisposition to macular degeneration, since her maternal grandfather is known to have had the disease. In addition, she adopted an unproven therapeutic technique that, along with the practice of not wearing sunglasses, may have contributed to her vision loss. Instead of allowing her diminished eyesight to stifle her artistic drive, she transferred her talents to alternative forms of art.

This artist's work has appeared in the most famous museums and art galleries and has been reproduced on posters and in calendars. Her overly large flowers force us to look closely at objects we would usually pay little attention to, and her landscapes have such gradations of color that they seem to be abstract design.

Although O'Keeffe (1887-1986) lived an active life

for ninety-nine years, at seventy-seven she experienced a sudden blurring of her vision while she was driving home on a particularly bright, sunny day. She had developed exudative, or wet, macular degeneration, which was complicated by a retinal vein blockage in her left eye. She continued her painting in spite of less than20/200 vision in each eye because, as she said, "I can see what I want to paint. The thing that makes you want to create is still there."

Casual observers felt that O'Keeffe appeared to function quite well despite her disability. Indeed, visitors would often observe that she seemed quite sure-footed along narrow paths and could identify specific mountains on the horizon. Of course, what those normal-sighted visitors failed to understand—as so many still do today—is that people with macular degeneration can make out general shapes in their surroundings while being unable to focus directly on the fine details.

While she was in her fifties, O'Keeffe developed a great enthusiasm for the work of Dr. W. H. Bates. In the 1930s, this eccentric ophthalmologist developed "eye exercises" that he described in the now-discredited book, *Perfect Sight Without Glasses*. In this book he advocated one exercise—looking directly at the sun while fluttering the eyelids—that we now know can be exceedingly damaging to the macula. O'Keeffe also refused to wear sunglasses in the dazzling New Mexico sun because she claimed it would distort the colors she saw. We cannot know with certainty whether these activities contributed directly to her macular degeneration, but there is now evidence that they certainly may have. In addition, because her grandfather had AMD, her case might have been one of genetic predisposition aggravated by repeated damage from ultraviolet light.

Seeing Things Anew

Few of us, of course, share the creative genius of O'Keeffe, Monet, and these other magnificent artists. But what we all have in common with them, and with each other, is the need to blaze our own trail of renewal. As with any personal journey, the biggest challenge often lies simply in finding the point of origin to that trail. The starting points are there. You just have to look beyond the clouds.

CHAPTER 14

Common Themes

All of us who have age-related macular degeneration have our own stories, our own vivid memories of how we first noticed our problem, our own experiences with doctors, our own ways of coping. Here are the stories of four of my acquaintances. Their names have been changed to protect their privacy.

Hank W.

Hank W., a former retailer, was sixty-two when he developed the wet type of macular degeneration.

YS: When did you first notice something was wrong with your vision?

HW: I was at a performance of the opera. You know how, when someone's head is in front of you, you move your own head slightly to the right or to the left so you can see the stage. When I moved my head to the right, such that I was viewing the stage with my right eye while my left eye was blocked by the person's head in front of me, everything was very clear.

But when I moved the other way, and I was seeing with my left eye, everything was fuzzy, like seeing it through a cloud. I couldn't believe what was happening. I went to an ophthalmologist and eventually was diagnosed with macular degeneration.

YS: What was your reaction at the time?

HW: Initially, I didn't think it was that serious. The doctor asked me if I had ever heard of macular degeneration. I hadn't. At that time it wasn't spoken about on television, as it is now. So he told me what it was. And he said, "I know you want to know if you're going to be blind. You're not going to be blind. You're going to be visually impaired." I didn't know exactly what to make of that. But I was concerned about whether it was going to affect the second eye. The first eye had already scarred, the bleeding had stopped, the scar had formed, so there was no treatment available for it. The damage had been done and it was finished. And I had some vision in that eye. The vision was impaired, but I was not sightless in that eye, and of course the other eye was fine.

YS: What happened next?

HW: I was very worried about the second eye becoming affected. My doctor told me there's about a 10 percent increased likelihood each year. In other words, after one year there's 10 percent likelihood, and the second year 20 percent, and so on. So it was pretty well guaranteed that in time the second eye would be affected. In fact it happened two years later. I had laser treatment, but it was not successful. It even may have ended up doing more harm than good. I don't know that to be a fact. I do know that the end result was not good. Eventually—not immediately, but eventually—my right eye hemorrhaged to the point where I lost all vision except light perception. I have no perception of normal light like daylight. If I stare at a ceiling light I could see that there was light emanating from there. So that's my right eye, and in my left eye, the first one that was affected, I have 20/400 vision.

YS: How does the scotoma, the blind spot, get in your way, and how do you work around it?

HW: It's not a spot as such; it's an irregular shape. In my day-to-day life I'm not conscious of the blind spot. The eye seems to fill in from your own imagination, from your own experience of what you knew when you could see well. It fills in that missing part, so if I stare at that picture frame and turn my eye in a certain way I know that I'm placing part of the picture frame in the blind area but my mind is filling it in for me. So I don't see it consciously as a picture frame with a dark area. The whole thing is visible to me, or maybe it's because I adjust the eye to what I'm looking at.

YS: Are you aware consciously of doing anything like that? Of what's called scanning, of moving your eye frequently or rapidly, to get images?

HW: I think it just comes as a reflex. Your eye discovers where it has to be to see anything. For example, I know that the way I'm facing, if I had the vision in my other eye you would be plainly visible to me. But right now I see your foot moving and your leg up to your knee but the rest of you doesn't exist, nor does anything else on the right side of me. But if I face around a little to put you within the range of this eye, I not only see you, I can see the piano and the plant.

YS: What about identifying people you know? Identifying someone's face can be very difficult.

HW: I have that problem. I often tell people I know very well that I can recognize you in a familiar environment where I expect you to be or where I know you are. But if I pass you in the street, I might never realize that it's you. I can't work around that. I can't recognize a person's face in an unfamiliar environment or where I wouldn't expect them to be. But I can recognize people I know in a familiar setting from a distance by their distinctive build, by their silhouette, by a certain contour of their head or body.

YS: How has it affected your life, your work, your relationships?

HW: It was a blow to give up driving. I've adjusted to the fact that I don't drive, but not being able to drive is definitely a handicap. To a large extent it is overcome by the fact that my wife can drive. The other thing was reading. I always carry a little magnifier with me. If I go to the supermarket I use the magnifier to read the dates on labels. With it I can read anything, it's just a chore. There is no way I can read for pleasure, but if I need to read something I can, either with the device that I eventually acquired, the closed-circuit TV, or with a magnifier. I still enjoy traveling. I can see the panorama, almost the same as a person with normal vision. What I can't see in the panorama is the detail that you would see with good vision. But I can see the mountains, the lakes, the forest. Of course, the colors of the leaves are jumbled.

YS: What about your independence?

HW: I've learned that the extent of your independence depends on your interests in life, what situation you're in, and what you can salvage out of it. I am able to salvage a great deal. I enjoy my life, I enjoy my kids, I enjoy my grandchildren and the activities and performances that we go to. I can ambulate, I can go out on the street by myself, I can go to the supermarket, to the bank by myself. I walk to the post office, which is a mile and a half. I cross my local streets without traffic control and I cross major streets with a traffic light. I can take a cab somewhere if my wife isn't available to drive me. I can do these things and I do these things. I don't dwell on the unfortunate part of the condition, because the unfortunate part of the condition is not overwhelming me. There are all degrees of blindness. I enjoy whatever independence I'm capable of, and it is a lot. I don't think that I've lost independence.

Abigail P.

Abigail P. developed severe macular degeneration in her sixties, and is now legally blind. She has had poor vision in one eye since infancy.

YS: How did you first notice your vision problem?

AP: It was on a Memorial Day weekend. Suddenly I couldn't see. I couldn't see the television. I couldn't see my medications to take them. I had someone drop me off at the doctor's office. He told me I have macular degeneration. When I walked out of there I had no idea where I was, because I had never been there before. I had figured I'd find a bus. But I couldn't even find my way off the curb. I was holding on to the lamppost, just standing there not knowing what to do. Finally some man who was waiting for his daughter to get through with her eye surgery at the eye center asked if he could help me. I said yes, I can't get home. So he took me back to the medical building and I had to ask someone to call a taxi for me.

YS: Can you describe your scotoma, the blind or hazy spot?

AP: Well, I can't see your face at all. I can see your body with my peripheral vision. One time I noticed that when I was having dinner the plate looked like it was broken, and I never break any dishes. I thought, "How on earth did that happen?" I put my hand on the plate to see what happened to it, and the plate was intact.

YS: How has it changed your life?

AP: Tremendously. My family is close, but we don't live near each other, so we talk on the telephone on weekends. My sisters come out on weekends; they took me food shopping. I appreciate it because I can't see the stuff on the shelves in the store.

YS: How do you ordinarily do your shopping?

AP: With difficulty. I used to walk thirteen blocks to the supermarket, but it's too dangerous for me to cross the big streets now. I was nearly hit by a big truck. It takes me about two hours to do my food shopping now; it used to take forty-five minutes. And only since I got my magnifying glasses a few weeks ago is it even doable. I can't even cut my nails. When I went into the clothing store, I couldn't see the clothing, I couldn't see the labels, I couldn't see the prices or the size. That I couldn't do such a personal thing, buy clothes, it just killed me.

YS: Sometimes even the most loving family or friends see you walking around the house, picking something up from the floor. They have no concept of the tremendous difficulty that AMD inflicts upon people. They may think you see better than you claim. Have you found this to be the case?

AP: They have no idea. They talk to me like I'm two years old. They don't understand. They think I'm worse than I am. They hold me by the hand to step down. I try to tell them that all I have to do is hold them by the arm, and when you're walking and you go down the step, I can feel that. But they don't understand that. I'd rather they didn't help me as much as they try to help me because all the help that they give me is wrong.

YS: In my practice I often see people who become somewhat depressed.

AP: I was not depressed, but I have had nightmares, especially at first. Successive nightmares, every night, the same dream. The nightmare was I was going to throw myself under a truck. I realize that was stupid; it was not my style. I told a few people about it and got it out of my system. And then the nightmares went away. But then when I lost the rest of my sight I was having bad nightmares again—being encased in something and screaming for help. You have to understand that I was always afraid of the dark, as a small kid and even as a grown-up. So obviously if I've been afraid of the dark all my life and I can't see—it just makes sense that I would be afraid and have nightmares.

YS: How do you deal with it?

AP: I'm more dependent on other people. I've gotten a lot of wonderful help from the Helen Keller Services for the Blind. Every single person has been extremely nice. They are totally trained and know before I tell them what I can't see. I like to be very self-sufficient. They gave me a guide to use so I can write checks. Around my house they put buttons on my microwave and on my stove. They gave me a little gizmo to put on my cup so it won't overflow. Before I got it, I was spilling things all over. They printed my recipes in large type so I can use them. I've managed to work around this myself for the most part.

Harold E.

Harold E., formerly a senior executive at one of the world's leading pharmaceutical companies, developed the wet type of macular degeneration in his early seventies.

YS: How did it all start with you?

HE: I was in the boardroom of my company one day, and people in my division had put up charts. I was looking at these charts and thinking that these guys did not make good charts today. There is something wrong; I can't see them. I said something about it and the doctor who was on the team told me I'd better go to see an ophthalmologist because the charts are wonderful. That's how I learned I had macular degeneration.

YS: What's been your experience with the doctors you've seen?

HE: Some have been quite good and others have not. Ten years after diagnosing my macular degeneration, my first retina specialist wanted to remove my cataracts. It turned out he hadn't been doing cataract surgery for many years and wasn't familiar with the newest procedures. I went to a very highly recommended retina specialist in London, who didn't even examine me. He just looked at the pictures of my eyes, and with his students around him told me I was going to go blind.

YS: He actually told you that you'd go blind?

HE: Yes, but after that I went to a marvelous doctor in Philadelphia. He gave me about a five-hour examination. And he told me, "Look, you'll never go blind. You'll walk into a room and see a figure; you won't be able to recognize the face. That's the worst that can happen to you, but you'll never go blind." Then I went to another specialist in New York. He was the most marvelous guy I've been to. He is so busy, but he gives his patients time. That's the thing that impressed me about him. The key to this condition is getting the right doctor who's interested in you, who will give you the time.

YS: How has your condition affected your lifestyle, your way of coping?

HE: I had to make a lot of adaptations. I use a closed-circuit television to read. I also use a stand magnifier. With my ordinary reading glasses I can read only with a lot of light. With the television machine, the smallest print I can read. It's beautiful. The low-vision aids have been very good for me. I went to the Lighthouse and they gave me special prism glasses and I've been using those quite successfully. My biggest problem is that my wife doesn't drive. If I can't drive I'm completely lost. I have a restricted license, and I only drive in a radius of five miles. I get the newspaper, I get bread, have a haircut, all in a five-mile radius.

YS: I find that with my patients, in my practice, episodes of depression are quite frequent. Have you had any similar problems?

HE: My depressions were very deep. I left New York City because I couldn't even see the traffic lights on the opposite side of the street. I couldn't go to shows anymore. I don't go to the movies anymore. I watch the television, but mostly I hear the television and I see some figures on it. It was an extremely depressing thing for me. Luckily I have a wonderful wife who's also a psychotherapist and who helps me a great deal. So I can live with it, get on with it, you know. I exercise; I live a simple life. I don't go out anymore if I can help it. I stay home, and I've gotten used to it. I've accepted it. I don't fight it anymore. I'm an optimist. I'm only hoping that something new will come up.

YS: What have you discovered on your own that seems to be of help to you?

HE: I've stopped drinking hard alcohol completely. I drink one glass of wine a day and that's all. And I exercise. I have a treadmill and I do one mile a day, and free-hand exercises for circulation and exercises for my back. I do these exercises five days a week.

YS: The other important factor, which many of my patients often mention, is family support.

HE: I'm very fortunate. My family understands my problem; in fact, they worry about me a great deal. They tell me to be careful, but I tell myself to be careful.

Ann R.

Ann R., a longtime homemaker, developed the wet type of AMD in her late sixties.

YS: When did you first notice you had a problem with your vision?

AR: I remember one time I was driving and I noticed that the yellow line, the dividing line, was absolutely wavy. I thought, "Oh my God, whoever painted that is crazy. Somebody didn't know what he was doing." I let it go, but it was strange, and then coming back, I noticed it again.

YS: After your diagnosis, what happened?

AR: I had laser treatment, and at first it was very successful. The day after the patch came off, I drove and the lines were straight! But then one day, early in the morning, I awakened and looked toward the hall where I always have a light, and I couldn't see it with my other eye, the right eye. It turns out I had a massive hemorrhage. It's been over a year since then, but I'm thrilled because I have wonderful peripheral vision, and now I can manage okay around the house.

YS: How did you feel when you first began to understand what was happening to your vision?

AR: Miserable—upset, of course. My first thought was "Oh, God! My world's turned upside down. I've lost my independence. I can't drive, I have to stay at home, I have to rely on everybody else for every little thing." And it really upset me quite a bit, especially the fact that I couldn't read. But then my daughter told me about this Aladdin closed-circuit TV system. I got it and it helps tremendously.

YS: What kinds of activities did you enjoy before you developed AMD that you can no longer

do, and how are you coping with this?

AR: I loved working outdoors and I loved all of nature so much. I loved projects. Reading. I loved to drive. I would drive out east to pick up my friends, and we'd go out and just look around the countryside and all. I used to love to cook, but I can't really cook now except maybe for bacon and eggs in the morning. I'll tell you one thing, I do find my way through a refrigerator.

YS: How did you find this affected your relationships with family and friends?

AR: I have wonderful friends who will call me and we will go to lunch together, so I do get about a bit. It's not easy because I was so independent and so active. My friends were wonderful. They really wanted to know if I needed anything or if I want to go somewhere. My grandsons are great. After they learned about what was happening to me, they said, "Nanny, we'll take care of you." That's wonderful, but I hate the word handicap, and I don't want people to grab my arm and hold me. I just don't want to be thought of as handicapped, because I feel I'm not.

YS: How have you reacted emotionally to this?

AR: There are days when I feel very blue. I get so frustrated; on occasion I find myself throwing something down and saying a not-nice word. It makes you feel better. But sometimes, however, there are moments—just moments—when I'll leave my bedroom and go to do something and I think: "Oh, God, just for a moment I forgot that I had this problem." It's such a wonderful feeling. It doesn't last long, but it's a great feeling. I used to think how horrible it must be to lose one's sight, and I could see this beautiful picture that used to go through my mind. The greens, the fruits, everything—all the wonderful color around me. Fortunately I can still see that. There are days when I am sitting here by myself and I think "Oh, heck!" and then I stop and say to myself, "It could be a lot worse. There are people far worse off than I am." Really, what more can one think?

CHAPTER 15

Low Vision Rehabilitation

As I discussed in chapter 10, the role of low vision rehabilitation has assumed a much more important part of helping people with AMD to resume a more normal life with greater independence and fulfillment. The American Academy of Ophthalmology, therefore, established a section on low vision rehabilitation with a prestigious committee of academics and clinicians who have dedicated their careers to research and clinical practice to help people with incurable visual impairment.

I have been privileged to serve on that committee and therefore can report to you a brief summary of an important ongoing project. Through the combined studies and efforts of dozens of experts nationwide, two related projects were launched under the title of "The SmartSight Initiative." This program was directed primarily to ophthalmologists and through them to their patients with AMD.

The material, designed for both the general ophthalmologist and the retinologist, was sent to every one of these specialists with two objectives. The first was to suggest new methods to evaluate levels of visual impairment and take the initial steps in helping their patients to overcome the handicap. The second objective was to establish criteria to refer patients to a low vision rehabilitation specialist.

Vision rehabilitation can help you make the most of your vision. When you first meet with a specialist in low vision rehabilitation be sure to ask these questions:

• Will the practitioner be able to provide you with a prescription for devices? Are some devices loaned before purchase or returnable?

• Will rehabilitation training include reading, writing, shopping, and cooking? Will lighting and glare be addressed?

Will there be a home and mobility assessment?

• Can the practioner offer referrals for resources and support groups?

• Are services billed to Medicare or other insurances? If not, what is the charge? (Medicare covers most services, but not devices.)

Here it may be helpful to present an interview I conducted with a renowned specialist in low-vision rehabilitation.

Janet DeBerry Steinberg, O.D., FAAO

Dr. Steinberg is the director of low-vision research and rehabilitation at the Scheie Eye Institute in Philadelphia.

YS: What should people understand about the objective of low-vision assistance?

JS: The objective of low-vision rehabilitation is to enable and empower people to perform their activities of daily living, whether it's reading, writing, or anything else. The goal is to help a visually impaired person function at a higher level.

YS: What is the most important ingredient to successful rehabilitation?

JS: The patient must have a willingness to change, a willingness to do things differently. For example, as you know, we can help someone read. If the patient wants to read we'll see to it that that patient can read. But the patient has to have a willingness to work with the doctor, to do things in a little bit different fashion, but in a very effective fashion. It's a matter of redirecting their thinking toward doing things differently.

YS: How do you open someone's eyes to the

need to accept change?

JS: By taking the blame away from the person and by putting it on the disease. The disease has caused the problem. You did not do anything to get here; you did not do anything wrong. For instance, with reading, it's important to understand that the disease has affected your eyes in such a way that you're just not going to be able to hold the reading material on your lap anymore, but you will certainly be able to read if you want to. The patient has to make the decision as to how important reading really is to them. If reading is important we can make it happen. But if it's not important, that is okay, too.

YS: Why is it so important not to postpone some sort of accommodation to these lifestyle changes?

JS: First, if you start early, then any lifestyle adjustments that you do have to make will come in smaller increments and will be easier to live with. Second, it gives you more time to deal with your vision loss, to make the necessary emotional adjustments. And third, and probably most important, you won't lose great gaps in your life. If someone has had difficulty reading from the time their vision went to 20/50 and I don't see them until they're 20/200, that's a big couple of years that they haven't been able to read. What does that mean to their ability to work, to their ability to enjoy life, to stay well-informed? Don't wait! Reclaim your life now!

YS: What's the best way for a patient to work with a low-vision specialist?

JS: It's what you should tell the low-vision specialist. "I want to be able to use a computer. I want to be able to read my prayer book. I want to be able to watch people go by on the street. I want to be able to see my grandchildren. I want to be able to pay my bills." What do you want to do? You need to get that message across. The whole approach of rehabilitation is goal oriented and goal specific. You've got to know what your goals are and state them clearly and immediately. If you can go in to the low-vision office and say, "I want to do this, this, and this," you're going to get ten times more help than if you say, "I want to see the way I used to." Realistically, that's not going to happen. What can happen is you can read, you can write, you can work, you can do your activities of daily living. We just have to learn what your priorities are and address your specific needs.

CHAPTER 16

Full Circle

The piece of eye tissue that we have been discussing throughout this entire book is somewhat smaller than the round end of an eraser on the back of a pencil. I find it frightening that so many of the glories of my world are dependent on this small dot of tissue. I am also still in awe of the complexity of the physical and chemical changes essential to accomplish what we all take for granted as normal seeing. But above all, I am profoundly grateful. After a lifetime in the study of medicine in general and of the eye in particular, I have read a great amount of literature and research on age-related macular degeneration. I must express my gratitude to all the scholars and clinicians who spent so much of their lives studying this vital little tissue island and its specific diseases. I hope for a breakthrough in the near future—not necessarily a cure for the disease, but some limits to its progression and perhaps even prevention of its onset in the very next generation.

It may be helpful here to review some of the key information presented in this book.

Nature of the Disease

Macular degeneration is the leading cause of legal blindness in people over age sixty-five in the United States, and in fact in all Western industrialized societies. The onset and progression of age-related macular degeneration varies greatly from individual to individual because AMD is really a broad spectrum of a disease, varying from a few large drusen with little decrease in vision to extensive scarring or bleeding under the macula. There has been a recent advance in the classification of the stages of both the wet and dry types of the disease. This should help in more accurate diagnosis and prognosis. It should also be of benefit in investigating the effectiveness of new treatments.

In all likelihood, AMD is a multifactorial disease, meaning it has several causes. Most likely, though, the basic susceptibility of the patient is genetic. This susceptibility is then acted upon, probably over many years, by environmental and nutritional factors that trigger the onset of the disease. Not only will further genetic research help identify those prone to AMD, but it will likely point to new therapies.

Drusen are the hallmark of macular degeneration. These are localized waste deposits that form in the tissue near or under the macula. These drusen may remain quietly in place and pose no danger, but if they increase in number and size and begin spreading, they can start the process of change that leads to macular degeneration. For instance, drusen can cause fine new blood vessels to develop under the macula that can leak fluid or blood, which causes the wet type of macular degeneration.

The wet form of the disease is the focus of most attention, even though it represents only about 10 percent of all AMD cases. This is because the wet form is sometimes treatable with anti-VEGF intraocular injections, photodynamic laser treatments, intraocular steroids or some combination of all three. The more prevalent dry form of the disease has no treatment, but it does progress quite slowly and generally does not lead to the same level of visual impairment as the wet form.

Major Risk Factors

Major risk factors for AMD include the following:

• *Gender.* It is more common among women.

• *Race.* It is much more common among whites than among African-Americans or Hispanics.

• *Genetics.* Most studies indicate a hereditary tendency.

• *Smoking.* This definitely appears related, possibly because of smoking's effects on the vascular system and perhaps because smoking decreases the amount of lutein, that sight-essential nutrient, in the human retina.

• *Hypertension.* There appears to be some relationship between high blood pressure and the development of AMD.

• *Body-mass index.* Being overweight has been associated with an increased incidence of AMD, particularly among men.

• *Light exposure.* Statistics are inconsistent, but seem to indicate that retinal changes may occur after long-term exposure to bright sunlight.

• *Nutritional deficiencies.* Diets low in antioxidants, such as vitamins C and E, and in nutrients such as lutein, zinc, and zeaxanthin, may contribute to the onset of AMD. These elements are important to the healthy functioning of the macula.

Rehabilitation

Although there is no cure now for age-related macular degeneration, there are techniques that everyone with low vision should adopt in order to function more independently and enjoy life more fully. These techniques can help, and they pose no risk. The basic principles are:

- Exactly correct glasses for distance

- Exactly correct glasses for near

- Instruction in proper illumination

- Adequate magnification

- Eccentric fixation (seeing with the edges of the macula)

- Utilizing nonoptical devices such as large-print books, felt-tipped pens, talking watches, scales, etc.

- Using closed-circuit TVs to enlarge anything with mini-video cameras

- Using reading machines, machines that scan and read back any printed material in a pleasant voice

Sorting It All Out

My own story has come full circle with this book. It started, as it does in so many people with age-related macular degeneration, with a very specifically remembered event. With me it was a missing part of a ceiling fan blade; with someone else it may have been bizarre curves in the white line in the middle of the road.

I am sure that my own despair, depression, and fear of loss of independence are no greater than those of any of my patients. What I may have excelled at, unfortunately, is an ability to cover up my feelings. I did well in hiding my emotions from friends and family—indeed, even from myself.

What I have learned is that the inability to reach out for help, a trait particularly common among men in our society, impedes the growth needed to overcome adversity. It also blocks one of the great gifts we can give to others: the opportunity to be of significant help to a person in need. When one person helps another, both the person in need and the helper benefit. A basic requirement for this ideal situation to occur, however, is the open statement of needs.

So, from the perspective of newly enlightened patient and doctor, I make several pleas:

The first plea is to my fellow ophthalmologists. Try to really feel the oppressive constancy of a central scotoma, a thick haze always in the way of everything and anything your patients really want to see. Take five minutes to sit quietly with your AMD patients and reassure them that you understand what they are dealing with, and that the disease will not result in the blindness that they fear. Emphasize to your patients that there are new and effective ways to overcome many of the difficulties they now face, and that the horizon is crowded with hopeful and encouraging prospects.

My second plea is to the family and friends of those whose life has been changed by this tiny circle of tissue. There is, in these relationships, a delicate balance between offering support and denying independence, between showing compassion and displaying pity. Listen to your loved one. Find out his or her true needs, and work in partnership to meet them constructively.

My last plea is to you, the patient. Although "seeing beyond the clouds" sounds like a lofty goal and difficult to reach, it is precisely the effort made that will place you there. This should be a new life where nonvisual rewards, finally recognized, will cause the scotomas to fade in importance as the richness of life's sensations, relations, and thoughts overwhelm you again in all their magnificence.

RESOURCES

Associations/Organizations/Foundations

American Academy of Ophthalmology
www.eyenet.org; P.O. Box 7424 San Francisco, CA 94120-7424; (415) 561-8500. Brochures and fact sheets on eye conditions and impairment.

American Council of the Blind
www.acb.org; 1155 15th St. NW, Suite 720 Washington, DC 20005; (800) 424-8666. National membership organization of the blind with state, local, and special interest chapters; free monthly magazine in large print and Braille, on cassette, and on IBM-compatible computer disk.

American Foundation for the Blind
www.afb.org; 11 Penn Plaza, Suite 300 New York, NY 10001; (800) 232-5463. National resource for people who are blind or visually handicapped.

American Macular Degeneration Foundation
www.macular.org; P.O. Box 515 Northampton, MA 01061; (413) 587-9475. Source for information on macular degeneration. Publishes newsletter; website contains bulletin board for people with macular degeneration.

American Printing House for the Blind
www.aph.org; 1839 Frankfort Avenue P.O. Box 6085 Louisville, KY 40206; (800) 223-1839. Large nonprofit organization devoted to providing special media tools and materials for the blind or visually handicapped persons.

Association for Education and Rehabilitation of the Blind and Visually Impaired
www.aerbvi.org; P.O. Box 22397 Alexandria, VA 22304; (703) 823-9690. Books and publications.

Better Vision Institute
www.bettervisioninstitute.org; 1800 North Kent St., Suite 1210 Roslyn, VA 22209; (800) 424-8422. Education on eye care.

Blinded Veterans Association
www.bva.org; 477 H St. NW Washington, DC 20001-2694; (800) 669-7079. Support programs and services for legally blind veterans for nonservice and service-connected visual impairment.

The Foundation Fighting Blindness
www.blindness.org; 11350 McCormick Road Hunt Valley, MD 21031; (888) 394-3937. National eye research organization funding research. Serves as a source of information for eye care specialists and affected people.

International Agency for the Prevention of Blindness
www.iapb.org; Room 6A03, Building 31 Bethesda, MD 20892; (301) 496-2234. Involved in worldwide effort to prevent and treat blindness.

Lighthouse International
www.lighthouse.org; 111 East 59th St. New York, NY 10022; (800) 829-0500. The world's leading resource on vision impairment. Advocacy and direct services programs further the goal of assisting people with vision loss to develop the skills they need, at home and in the workplace, to lead productive independent lives.

Macular Degeneration Foundation Education, Inc.
www.eyesight.org; P.O. Box 9752 San Jose, CA 95157; (888) MDF-EYES. Offers information, counseling, and support for patients with AMD and their families.

Macular Degeneration International
www.maculardegeneration.org; 6700 North Oracle Road, Suite 505 Tucson, AZ 85704; (520) 797-2525. Publishes news journal of medical research and low vision rehabilitation. Sponsors seminars for the public.

National Association for Visually Handicapped
www.navh.org; 22 West 21st St., 6th Floor New York, NY 10010; (212) 889-3141. Offers extensive support services for the visually handicapped.

National Eye Institute

www.nei.nih.gov; 31 Center Dr. MSC 2510 Bethesda, MD 20892-2510; (301) 496-5248. Provides publications on eye diseases and information on current eye research.

National Federation of the Blind

www.nfb.org; 1800 Johnson St. Baltimore, MD 21230; (410) 659-9314. National advocacy organization with local chapters of partially sighted and blind members. Offers magazine and other print materials in large print and Braille and on cassette. Maintains referral and job services.

Prevent Blindness America

www.preventblindness.org; 500 East Remington Rd. Schaumburg, IL 60173; (800) 331-2020. Organization publishes educational materials on blindness.

Large-Print Publishers

Doubleday Large Print Home Library

www.doubledaylargeprint.com; P.O. Box 6325 Indianapolis, IN 46206; (800) 688-4442. Provides hardcover editions of best-sellers in large print, and a large-print book club.

New York Times Large Print Weekly

http://homedelivery.nytimes.com/; 229 W. 43rd St. New York, NY 10036; (800) 631-2580. Large-type version of The New York Times.

Reader's Digest/Large Type Edition
https://www.rd.com/offer/rdlp/giftown03/index.jsp
P.O. Box 241 Mount Morris, IL 61054; (800) 877-5293
Offers subscription to Reader's Digest, condensed books, Great Biographies series and the Bible in large print.

Thorndike—G.K. Hall Large Print Books
P.O. Box 159 Thorndike, ME 04986; (800) 257-5157. Large-print books; call or write for catalogue.

Ulverscroft Large Print, Inc.
www.ulverscroft.co.uk; P.O. Box 1230 West Seneca, NY 14224-1230; (800) 955-9659. Provides direct sale of large-print books.

The World at Large, Inc.
1689 46th St. Brooklyn, NY 11204; (800) 285-2743. Bi-weekly large-print newspaper with articles from news-magazines.

Xavier Society for the Blind
www.xaviersociety.com; 154 E. 23rd St. New York, NY 10010; (800) 637-9193. Free large-print Bibles for the blind and visually impaired.

Audiotapes

AudioBooks Online
www.audiobooksonline.com; RR 1, Box 60 Richmond, VA 05477; (802) 434-5550. Sells audio books online.

Aurora Ministries/Bible Alliance
www.auroraministries.org; P.O. Box 621 Bradenton, FL 34206; (941) 748-3031. Audio Bibles free to patients with certificate of visual, impairment.

Blackstone Audio Books
www.blackstoneaudio.com; P.O. Box 969 Ashland, OR 97520; (800) 729-2665. Audio books for rental or purchase.

Books on Tape
www.booksontape.com; P.O. Box 7900 Newport Beach, CA 92658 (800) 626-3333. Audio books

Media Access Group
www.wgbh.org/dvs; 125 Western Ave. Boston, MA 02134; (800) 333-1203. National service that makes PBS-TV programs, Hollywood movies, video, and other visual media accessible to people who are blind or visually impaired.

Library of Congress
www.loc.gov/nls; National Library Service for the Blind 1291 Taylor St. NW Washington, DC 29542; (800) 424-8567. Books and magazines on audiotape.

Recording for the Blind and Dyslexic
www.rfbd.org; 20 Roszel Rd. Princeton, NJ 08540 Nationwide lending library for the blind and visually handicapped.

Tools for Independent Living

Abledata
www.abledata.com; 8455 Colesville Rd., Suite 935 Silver Spring, MD 20910; (800) 346-2742. Products, services, and information on assisted technology and rehabilitation equipment.

Ann Morris Enterprises
www.annmorris.com; 890 Fams Court East Meadow, NY 11554; (800) 454-3175. Low-vision products.

Benetech
www.benetech.org; P.O. Box 215 Moffett Field, CA 94035; (800) 444-4443. Nonprofit organization providing low-vision reading systems and devices.

Associated Services for the Blind
www.asb.org; 919 Walnut St. Philadelphia, PA 19107; (215) 627-0600. Provides low-vision products and services for the blind and visually handicapped.

Big Type Company
www.bigtypeco.com; 4701 W. Mill Rd. Milwaukee, WI 53218; (800) 933-1711. Large-print address books, calendars/ check registers, notebooks.

Can-Do Products
www.independentliving.com; 27 East Mall Plainview, NY 11803; (800) 537-2118. Low-vision products.

Captek Science Products

www.captek.net; P.O. Box 888 Southeastern, PA 19399; (800) 888-7400. Low-vision aids, recreation products, electronic products, large print, toys and games.

Carolyn's Products for Enhanced Living

1415 57th Ave. West Bradenton, FL 34207; (800) 648-2266. Low-vision products.

Dolphin Computer Access LLC

www.yourdolphin.com; 100 South Ellsworth Ave., 4th floor San Mateo, CA 94401; (650) 348-7401. Sells computer screen readers, screen magnifiers, OCR programs, Braille translation systems, and speech synthesizers for computers.

General Electric Corporation

Consumer Affairs; Appliance Park, Louisville, KY 40225; (800) 626-2000. Tactile knobs for electric appliances and overlays for microwave and washer/dryer units.

G.W. Micro

www.gwmicro.com; 725 Airport North Office Park Fort Wayne, IN 46825; (219) 489-3671. Computer software and hardware solutions for blind and visually impaired people.

Innoventions, Inc.

www.magnicam.com; 5921 South Middleheld Rd., Suite 102 Littleton, CO 80123; (800) 854-6554. Source of the Magni-Cam, a portable, affordable electronic magnifier for people with low vision.

L.S.&S. Group

www.lssproducts.com; P.O. Box 673 Northbrook, IL 60065; (800) 468-4789. Low-vision and hearing-impaired products.

Massachusetts Association for the Blind

www.mablind.org; 200 Ivy St. Brookline, MA 02446; (800) 682-9200. Products and services for blind and visually impaired people.

Maxi Aids

www.maxiaids.com; 42 Executive Blvd. Farmingdale, NY 11735; (800) 522-6294. Low-vision products.

MONS International, Inc.

www.magnifiers.com; 6595 Roswell Rd., Suite 224 Atlanta, GA 30328; (800) 541-7903. Sells Braille watches, Optelec CCTVs, games, talking calculators, four-track recorders, kitchen aids, writing guides, magnifiers, computer software and accessories, greeting cards, talking scales, etc.

NoIR Medical Technologies

www.noir-medical.com; 6155 Pontiac Trail South Lyon, MI 48178; (800) 521-9746. Sunglasses for ultraviolet and infrared protection.

Telecom Pioneers

www.telecompioneers.org; P.O. Box 13888 Denver, CO 80202; (800) 976-1914. Has local chapters that manufacture various products for visually impaired persons.

Telesensory Corporation

www.telesensory.com; 520 Almanor Ave. Sunnyvale, CA 94086; (800) 227-8418. Produces low-vision systems and other high-tech devices for the visually impaired.

Vision World Wide, Inc.

www.visionww.org; 5707 Brockton Dr. Indianapolis, IN 46220; (800) 431-1739. Offers informative magazine and referral help line.

LowVision.com

www.lowvision.com; 3030 Enterprise Ct., Suite D., Vista, CA 92081; (800) 826-4200. Comprehensive line of low vision solutions, daily living products, video-magnifiers and optical products.

The Amsler Grid

Amsler grid testing can serve as a useful early warning test for macular degeneration, especially the wet form. Patients with the dry form of the disease should use the Amsler grid regularly to provide an early warning of a possible onset of the wet form of the disease.

To use the Amsler grid, hold it at a normal reading distance and then stare at the central spot, first with one eye closed and then the other. Be sure to wear your reading glasses if you use them. Continue staring at the central dot while paying attention to the surrounding lines. If any of the lines appear wavy, bent, gray, or fuzzy, or are absent in certain areas of the grid—or if you cannot see the central dot—consult your ophthalmologist.

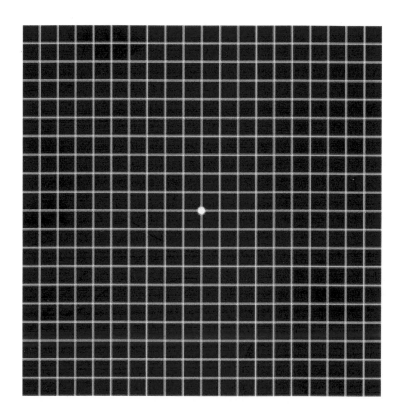

Glossary[*]

Bruch's membrane A thin layer of retinal tissue separating the retinal pigment epithelium from the choroid.

Choroid The vascular, pigmented tissue layer between the sclera and the retina. It provides the blood supply for the outer retinal layers.

Cornea The transparent front "window" of the eye that serves as a major refractive surface.

Drusen Yellow-white waste deposits found in Bruch's membrane, generally increasing with age and almost always associated with age-related macular degeneration.

Fluorescein angiography A technique for examining the retina that involves the injection of a harmless fluorescing dye in the arm and then photographing the effects of the dye as it reaches the retinal blood vessels.

Fovea The oval depression in the center of the macula.

---

[*] Definitions of ocular anatomy are adapted from *The Physician's Guide to Eye Care,* by Jonathan D. Trobe, M.D. (American Academy of Ophthalmology, 1993) and *Basic Ophthalmology,* by Cynthia A. Bradford, M.D. (American Academy of Ophthalmology, 1999).

Free radicals Molecules made unstable by a change in their atomic structure, typically as a result of oxidation. Chemical reactions caused by free radicals can lead to a variety of harmful effects in the body, including damage to the cells of the macula.

Lens The transparent pea-sized body suspended behind the pupil and iris; part of the refractive mechanism of the eye.

Macula The area of the retina at the posterior pole of the eye responsible for fine, central vision.

Optic disc The portion of the optic nerve visible within the eye. It is comprised of axons whose cell bodies are located in the ganglion cell layer of the retina.

Oxidation The chemical process by which cells use oxygen to create energy.

Pupil The circular opening in the center of the iris that adjusts the amount of light entering the eye.

Retina The neural tissue lining the back of the eye. Essentially transparent except for the blood vessels on its inner surface, the retina sends the initial visual signals to the brain via the optic nerve.

Retinal pigment epithelium The outermost layer of the retina.

Rods and cones The light-sensing nerve cells of the retina.

Sclera The thick outer coat of the eye, normally white and opaque.

Scotoma Blind spot. In patients with age-related macular degeneration, it usually takes the form of a translucent, cloudy patch in the central part of the visual field.

Visual acuity A measurement of the smallest object a person can identify at a given distance from the eye.

Vitreous cavity The relatively large space (4.5 cc) behind the lens that extends to the retina. The cavity is filled with a transparent jelly-like material called vitreous humor.

3791367

Made in the USA